PART 1

Did you ever stand by the side (
stranger's baby in a pram? Did you ever listen to the instructions in your head, to take the pram and push it under a lorry? Did you ever think these thoughts were nothing to do with you at all? That they'd been implanted in your head by powerful, malevolent entities? Did you ever think, 'I've got to do this ... I've got no choice?

Did you ever?

CHAPTER 1 ADRIFT

I was adrift as soon as I arrived in that unfamiliar northern town. But I didn't know it, and I hadn't the faintest idea of what was to come. I'd like to reach back and shake that young woman. 'Just walk away,' I'd say. 'Cut your losses, it's not the end of the world.' Does she really not know that time is running out?

When did it all start? I'll begin with what I thought was the beginning. It's a totally unremarkable scenario. There's me sitting on the bed, in my newly rented flat, one afternoon in November 1998. New flat, new job, new life. I'm a museum curator. It's not long after my thirtieth birthday, a milestone, 'have you got it all together?' sort of age. Well, I knew I fell short in some ways, but I wasn't doing too badly overall.

The removal men wouldn't be here until tomorrow, as they had 200 miles to come. They had collected everything that morning; friendly blokes who had asked me, 'Do you recognise us? We were on that TV programme: *Neighbours from Hell*. We moved the lady next door.' The answer was 'no', and it was an odd sort of reference, but I could see we were a match. They had a beat up white van and I had beat up possessions. They complained about the weight of the old settee from the gallery, calling it a 'lump' with its cast iron frame. They'd had to carry it up the steps from my old basement flat. I didn't tell them that they'd have to carry it up the steps again when they arrived.

This was a much nicer flat altogether, totally unlike the damp dirty basement I had lived in before, where if you left books on the floor they sucked up the water from the clay underneath and soon became wrinkled. I had raided skips for old bricks and scaffolding wood to build makeshift shelves. My then colleagues had been too polite to say anything, but I suspected I always smelled of mushrooms. It would have made a good subject for Nick Hedges and his Shelter camera, but I was resilient enough.

That scabrous and unsavoury flat was, however, home. I planted window boxes of red geraniums and kept the yard tidy. The student litterers, who saw the basement entrance of my home as a handy bin for bottles, crisp packets and chips in curry sauce, were infuriating, but their rubbish could be collected and binned. It was controllable. I harassed the rat that moved in under the steps, probably a refugee from a nearby building project, so it soon left for somewhere less stressful. My friends occasionally referred to the flat as, 'the serial killer's basement,' but, thanks to me, it presented a respectable front to the world and, serial killing aside, it was still a benign environment in spite of noisy students overhead.

However, this new flat was totally different. I was earning more money and property in this town was cheaper. The flat was in a reasonable quality, historic building that had been properly converted, and it was dry, light and relatively spacious. I found the cold wintry light shocking after living in subterranean gloom. It was a strange white atmosphere that left me nowhere to hide, and the whiteness and strange sense of frost was compounded by, as I soon discovered, malfunctioning heating.

There were letters for me already. My new employers had sent me a thick white envelope of paperwork. More frost. I picked it up nervously, then opened it and forced myself to sit and look through it. Upcoming exhibition projects were listed and I soon noticed that my name, as the project lead, was mentioned again and again; in fact, it seemed, more than anyone else. It was a disquieting read. These projects had been envisaged by other people, yet it was me who'd have to creatively realise them. It didn't occur to me that I could have, and should have, negotiated a less alarming workload. These were only museum exhibitions after all, hardly crucial. Nobody would die (or even be slightly hurt), if they didn't happen quite as planned. But I had been a junior assistant previously, and that was how I still thought. I was accustomed to being told what to do.

This paperwork, I believed, clearly laid out what I was expected to achieve in my new, more responsible role as curator of decorative arts (that's antiques rather than paintings), so I needed to pull myself together and get on with it. 'Not fair, not fair,' I thought, and felt desperate, childish tears building up inside me - but I wasn't a child; I was a grown up. I'd chosen to move here; nobody but me had precipitated this life change. Nobody had picked me up and dropped me here, for obscure reasons of their own.

What had I done? It was one thing to impress an interview panel with bold talk and promises, but it was quite another to produce the confident, intelligent and successful person I'd sold them. Could I deliver? Had I sold them a lie? I didn't lie on my CV; I was qualified to do the job. I had the relevant experience and qualifications, but did I really have the personal qualities I advertised? Would the job be one long round of compensation: 'I'm sorry, I know who I am, I'm sorry you've got me ... I didn't mean to, I don't know what I was thinking.'

Did I even really want to be here? Had I only applied for the new job because everybody expected me to? Perhaps I should have done more thinking before I applied. In my previous job I was a sheltered junior, where all the real responsibility was processed and allocated by a senior curator. I was happy there; I had friends and was well supported. I didn't want to leave, and had gone through the rituals of leaving - the meal, the present, the signature-filled card, while suppressing anxious and sentimental tears, and pretending to be happy and excited. I had felt obliged to leave, once I was offered this new job - silly really, because I wasn't the only applicant. It might have been better to walk away.

Now, I had to face reality: the 'getting a new job' game was over. I had been busily playing it while carefully avoiding the implications, but I couldn't avoid it any longer. I was committed to my new life as an unsheltered grown-up, visible on my own merits, and it all felt very wrong, but not fatally wrong - at least not yet. After all, I was hardly inexperienced when it came to moving about and creating a new life for myself. I'd been to an unfamiliar city for university, and my last job had been in another, previously unknown, city. This time, however, it was different. Previously, I had wanted to be in those new places. Now I didn't, but at least I did know how to gently uncurl myself into a new environment, and how to gradually map out the safe spaces and build them into the architecture of my brain. It was never easy; as a timid person I always had to push myself on, but weakness could be overcome with mental discipline and positivity. Anybody could do anything … it had worked so far for me, so it was going to work again. That was not negotiable.

So, I got off the bed and went outside to sort out the structural components of my new life.

It was wintry, but not a bad day, chilly and sunny. Even on a weekday afternoon, the town was busy but towns *were* busier in those days before internet shopping. I found the laundrette, the bank, the nearest supermarket, and I bought a new washing up bowl from Woolworths. At some point, I bought a cylinder vacuum cleaner, bright red, and made by Goblin. The name was very unsuited to the product. My mother liked bright red kitchenware and appliances, from her red-handled scissors to her tomato soup coloured AGA, so the colour was mildly reassuring, reminding me of a safe, loving upbringing and a certain lightness of being.

As I walked through the shopping streets, I tried to be invisible, vaguely hoping that if I was invisible, I was not really there - that I was really a sort of transitory ghost from somewhere else, a 'somewhere else' that was my real home. Not this place. I blocked my ears to the new and unfamiliar, local accent; people here spoke more loudly, and they were friendlier in the shops. I didn't mind their friendliness, but I didn't want to engage with it, to accept that my invisible ghostly presence was solid and real to these people, that to them I really existed. If I could have navigated the outside world with my eyes shut, I would have done so, but I had to see the red brick buildings, and the sloping streets. They were strikingly different, as I had just come from a flat, stone-built city. I could pretend that I was not here in this town, but I'd know it was a pretence. I was here, every part of me. It was my new reality.

I forced myself to go and look at my new place of work, so I could time how long it would take to walk there from the flat. This would be my new working day routine. I liked to live within walking distance of work, as it gave me total autonomy over my schedule and I didn't have to worry about public transport. The museum was one of the grandest buildings in the town, Victorian high drama at its best, and its beauty and quality was comforting. I knew I could learn to love this building. Perhaps, I could learn to love this new life. I had gossamer-thin hope, but hope nonetheless. It was just a case of doing things properly. It was just a case of believing and counting my blessings. I had lots of blessings, so that was a good starting point.

CHAPTER 2 JUST TRY HARDER

My new life didn't start too badly. I might not have wanted to be here, but it was easy to make the best of things. There were so many positives to this job. My new colleagues were congenial and friendly, I was treated fairly and pleasantly, the job was interesting, and it was what I had trained to do. Away from work, the town was large, had good railway connections and property was cheap, so everything looked promising for getting out and about and exploring this new environment. I was fortunate, and I knew it.

I actively engaged with the job and worked on several projects. My future was in this town; perhaps I'd stay here for the rest of my working life. I had no desire (or aptitude) to go into management, and the pay was ample for my unambitious lifestyle. It should be easy, I thought, to master this new life and shape it into a mould that suited me.

This was not a time to bury my talents; instead I needed to use them - to nurture them, to be a success, and this success would boost my confidence and performance. That is how a good life works; it should be a cycle of positive reinforcement. I knew all that stuff, as I'd listened to the *Parable of the Talents* at least a hundred times, in dull school assemblies. That was as motivational as my school got in the 1980s. I recently visited a secondary school hall and noticed it was festooned with uplifting and inspiring quotes - not that I knew any of them, there was certainly nothing biblical nowadays. Anyway, I'd always felt some sympathy for the least able man who buried his master's talent. He still had that talent to dig up when his master returned. It had been safely looked after, so why was his master so ungrateful? That servant's self-confidence had already been fatally undermined by his master, when he received the least number of talents to look after in the first place.

Outside work, I explored the town. I soon discovered the large, central park, happily only a short walk away. It was an attractive and entertaining Victorian inheritance, with a Japanese garden, a lime tree walk by the river, a grand fountain and large plant-filled urns. My flat was gardenless. I didn't even have access to the rear yard, so visiting this park was an especial, escapist delight, a small window into a beautiful and spiritually refreshing world. The area nearest the park had a wistful Georgian grace, a reminder of when the town was a fashionable destination. Later, it became an industrial town thickly seeded with mills, workshops and row upon row of modest terraced houses. Now, it was a post-industrial town; the surviving mills were mostly vacant and, over the years, the town planning department had busily chipped away at the terraced rows. It gave the town a skeletal, disjointed air, somewhat forlorn and knocked about.

The man in the flat next door was friendly. We went out for walks and he told me useful things. 'Don't swim in the river near that bridge,' he said, although I had no plans to do so, 'Lots of people have drowned there.' I imagined a long line of local residents, swept away by this hostile river and spat out into the Irish Sea. He showed me parts of the town I might not have gone to otherwise. We looked at the old docks, now reimagined with shops and flats; an odd place, surrounded by tall, flat buildings. I found it windswept and bleak and wouldn't have wanted to live there, but I don't like open bleak places anyway. They make me watch my back.

My new friend was a poet, and informed me he was always thinking and creating, as poetry takes a huge amount of mental effort. I said, 'Oh yes,' politely, fully aware that I was a poetry philistine. My tastes are childish, in spite of an English A-level, and I rarely read poetry. I like Edward Lear, John Betjeman and, especially, Robert Herrick:

The Hag is astride,

This night for to ride;
The Devill and Shee together ...

This Herrick poem has me anxiously, and surreptitiously, glancing at the Halloween night sky, hoping not to see a storm-tossed witch. Not a very adult response ...

One afternoon, we ventured over the river downstream and ended up in a quiet, deserted park. He was struggling with a poem and sat for a long time, on a park bench, looking anguished, while I made a few suggestions. 'You could try a semicolon?' I offered. My helpful suggestions were clearly unwanted, so he separated himself from me and positioned himself under a tree with his back to me, apparently contemplating the view but rather, I suspected, to make a point. I continued to sit on the bench and gazed at the pink, spring blossom. It was the obvious inspiration for a Japanese haiku but I didn't know how to write one. There was nothing else to do: it was boring, cold and awkward. Was I supposed to abandon him and go home? I wished I understood poetry and didn't have such a pedestrian and unimaginative mind. I was clearly never going to be a poetic muse, as I was not overcome with passionate admiration for the creative process and was obviously far too impatient. He eventually relented. I never knew if he'd fixed the troublesome line, but I was left with the feeling that I had somehow managed to sabotage his creativity.

It was an on and off friendship, and after a few months he fell out with me for the first time. He was fundamentally a kind man, but it was clear to both of us that we had differing values. I believed, unless you were ill, you shouldn't live on benefits. He believed that, unless he was supported by benefits, he couldn't realise his full creative potential. I wondered whether if he had a more outgoing life he might have found his creativity enriched and easier to access. He was adamant that there was no way he could do any job other than some creative writing tutoring, and that the kind of jobs I had done, and was prepared to do, were not suitable for him (but obviously fine for me). Presumably, I was made from baser clay. He was probably right, but there was part of me that wondered if this was a good use of my taxes.

Immediately after what appeared to be a pleasant, uneventful walk, he wrote me a letter and pushed it under the door. It was a nasty shock as it described, at length, what a ghastly, arrogant person I was. I felt some compunction as I had probably been impatient with him. Had I perhaps looked down on him, seeing him as little more than a friendly, local tour guide, with time on his hands? That must be what he believed and this was his hurt revenge. Even so, what had I done that was so dreadful? Why had I caused such an explosion of hate? Who wrote letters like this on a pretty card anyway? Poets, obviously. I'd never met one before. It was a sugared bomb, so I threw it away, nobly resisting the urge to slide a letter under his door inscribed, 'Same to you with knobs on …,' or something equally inelegant. It was a painful reminder of my environmental dissonance, my fundamental lack of belonging. Nothing like this had happened in my previous life.

However, there was increasingly less time now for undirected walking about the town, as I was busier and busier at work. This new preoccupation was chiefly of my own making. In spite of all my good intentions, I couldn't relax into my new, good life. I continued to persevere when, perhaps, I should have cut and run. I was working to the basic principle that if things were not right, I was clearly not trying hard enough. So, I tried harder and harder, and became increasingly melancholic, self-absorbed, and conscience ridden.

Unfortunately, I'd walked into a delicate situation in my new workplace, and delicate tact isn't one of my strengths. I learned that a junior colleague had applied for my job and didn't get it. It was awkward for both of us and the embarrassment drove me on; there was absolutely no way I was going to justify his grievances. I had to outperform him. Some of my new colleagues supported me, some of them supported him. There was an obvious and uncomfortable fault line in the office. My new, morbid consciousness worried about what my new manager and colleagues might think. Perhaps they already regretted employing me, when they could have had him. This junior colleague shared my projects in the early days; the aim was to help him feel better. I don't know if it did but it certainly didn't make me feel better. I felt like a usurper, and he clearly disliked me, but I'm not sure if under any circumstances we would have been friends.

As I felt my confidence slowly slipping away, I fantasised about other lifestyles. Anything and everything. I even considered contacting a couple of men from my past and asking someone to father a baby with me. Not only would I have loved to be a mother, but then I would have some real, vital concerns, and I could escape my unhealthy obsession with work. But it wasn't a realistic idea, however tempting. These poor men weren't some kind of baby shopping channel, waiting for my business. The idea was bizarre. What about their partners? There was no way I would have a baby without a steady relationship. My desire for motherhood couldn't outweigh a child's welfare. It was a selfish, irresponsible idea. The baby would be solely reliant on me. What if something happened to me? What if the baby was a boy? How could I be a father to a boy? Did I really think I'd be a good mother, or was I just looking for a get-out clause?

I wished that I'd been able to build long term relationships and wasn't such a freak. I'd had boyfriends but my anxiety would always push them away. I could never escape the memory of the unwanted maulings of my teenage years. It hurt these rare, later lovers who were gentle and undemanding. I made victims of them, so I gave up on love on the grounds that I wasn't really suited to a trusting relationship. But that still didn't stop me thinking about men, and longing for male love and company. How much easier life would be, I thought, if I didn't have to face everything alone.

Things didn't get better, but I persevered, against all my

gut instincts, and started house hunting. This was something I had been really looking forward to. I'd had enough of rented properties: landlords who kept deposits, broken appliances, never being able to change anything, and living in perpetual uncertainty. I was sure that the stability and mental comfort of home ownership would help with the job, and sorting out my own home would be a creative distraction too. I would also feel more a part of the town. My southern accent made me an instant outsider every time I spoke, but once I'd bought into the fabric of the place, surely I would feel more psychically integrated.

It was before the age of property websites, so each week I inspected the property pages in the local paper and trailed shyly round the local estate agents. I could afford something quite large in the central areas, perhaps a six bedroom terrace or a picturesque ruin, but I was realistic enough. I didn't want to spend a lot of money and there were plenty of nineteenth century small, red brick terraced houses available. Although I could drive, I didn't own a car and had no plans to buy one, so I wasn't worried about parking. Neither did I have to consider schools, or indeed anybody else's requirements. As usual, it was just me.

It was late spring, then summer, and my house hunting coincided with a run of fine Saturdays. For the first time, I objectively and minutely observed the town's housing stock. I was brought up in a chalk area, where basements are rare and the small, older houses sit almost foundationless on their stable, chalk bases. This northern town was built on old shifting clay and it was not unusual for houses to be lopsided. At worst, you could see bricks sticking out like zip teeth from facades, and in a few other houses the floors sloped dramatically. These houses, according to the local estate agents, were, 'in need of some cosmetic redecoration,' as if Dulux paint had some kind of magical, stabilising properties. The sloping houses made me nervous; I could sense them shifting beneath my feet. Anything on castors would have to be propped against the lowest wall, and the old trick of removing a tablecloth from underneath a china tea service would be pointless. The tea service would slide off anyway; a slight exaggeration, but that's how it felt.

Surely, buying a house would be fun? It was only a form of shopping on a grand scale, but it was far more complicated than I had realised. This town was new to me, so I didn't have inbuilt layers of local knowledge. I had to compensate with visual checklists. Did the neighbours have bars on their windows? Perhaps not here, then ... Was the house right next door to one of the tower block estates where, every time I sat in my yard, I would be observed by hundreds of potentially alarming people? Was it down by the river? The riverside area was attractive but I could see large concrete flood defences. What would happen if they weren't big enough? Would I spend my life dreading heavy rain, and mentally assessing how many hours of safety were left before I was paddling in the front room? And then, of course, 'Oh so **this** is the local red light district ...'

Then there were the vendors. I soon realised that some people didn't really want to sell their houses at all. After viewing one immaculate house, I was informed that I was not 'suitable' for the property. There was no explanation for my lack of suitability, and part of me speculated that I should have admired the Mies van der Rohe style recliner in the Victorian front room - or maybe, more likely, the vendor wanted a cash buyer for a quick sale. At another house, I arrived at 10am, knocked on the front door and was told firmly by the semi- wrecked, hostile tenants that the house was not for sale. At least my knock had let some fresh air into their house, which reeked of cigarettes, weed, and alcohol. I had no desire to be caught up in a row between a landlord and his tenants. What if the tenants refused to go? Would we all end up living together? Our lifestyles didn't look to be at all compatible. Another dead end.

There really was so much to consider. How close was it to work, to the station, to the shops? Did the neighbours look OK? Were they students? I'd had enough of noisy students, cheerfully awake at 2am, and silent as the grave when I was getting up early for work. The longer I searched, the more the apparently limitless stock of small, red terraced housing possibilities diminished, as my requirements turned out to be far more exacting than I'd originally anticipated. I soon realised that I wasn't searching for the perfect house; I was searching for a perfect street.

At last I found a house, in a perfect street, close to the town centre. It was tightly hemmed in by main roads and scrappy, partially demolished streets, so the contrast was startling when I came across this tranquil and harmonious dolls' house square. The modest, neat, red brick terraced houses were tidily positioned around a church and presbytery. The church was stone-built, large and magnificent, and it dominated the square, with the little red houses clustered round its feet like courtiers. The town planners, so busy in the immediate area, had decided to leave the square untouched and now the houses were listed. The square was a tiny conservation area all by itself. It had been suspended in time. Nobody, now, could break its gentle rhythm.

On this beautiful, sunny Saturday morning, the square was quiet. The people who lived here weren't rich but they were respectable and their houses were reasonably well kept. At first glance, the houses looked identical, but they had actually been built in sections over a number of years and there were minor differences in the facades. The house I was viewing that day was on the west side of the square, the nicer side, where each house had two upstairs windows and one downstairs, to the right of the front door. The lintel over the front door was supported by modest corbels. There was a small front garden with an iron gate, so you could hear people coming in and out. The street was a dead end, terminating with a primary school, a metaphorical repository of innocence. I looked forward to hearing the children in the playground; it was a sound I'd always enjoyed.

I decided then, that whatever the condition of the inside, I would purchase this house. I was going to buy into this tranquil, dream-like square. It contained the first real peace I'd found in the town, but, I had to admit, the interior of the house didn't really live up to the exterior. It had been enthusiastically part-

modernised and it was definitely scruffy. However, internal issues could always be fixed, unlike the external environment.

It was a slightly distracted viewing, as the vendors' large family dog followed me about, licking my legs. I don't mind dogs, but I was surprised they didn't call him off. Perhaps, I said it was all right; I can't remember. The sellers apologised that the sash windows hadn't been replaced because of the listing, and I assured them that this really wasn't an issue. I was secretly glad. Overall, the house didn't seem to be particularly damp and the floors felt level. The facade looked level too. There were some alarming cracks inside, and the surveyor later informed me that the whole house was leaning backwards, but it had been like this for many years and was unlikely to move any further. I set about the business of buying, relieved I didn't have to face any more viewings.

This was partly because the viewings had been eating into my work schedule, and at work I could feel things slipping through my fingers. I was confused, unhappy and generally unsettled. If I didn't want to be living here, and more to the point shouldn't be here, then why was I buying a house? Was it just because everyone expected me to, and I didn't want my family and friends to glimpse my problems? The problems that I shouldn't have, anyway.

I seemed to be industriously spinning a web and, at the same time, transforming myself into a great, struggling fly. A deeply duplicitous fly, as I lied to friends and relatives. 'Yes, it's really good, thanks, I'm buying a house ...' People believed my fiction as it all sounded perfectly reasonable. So, why couldn't I live this fiction? My fictional reality was a good place to be, wasn't it?

CHAPTER 3 NEW FRIENDS

My house-buying was an act of bravado, as I was increasingly caught up in my own dreary psychodrama. My self-loathing was becoming brutal. I'd done my best to mould myself to this new life but I hadn't succeeded. I could have understood if something nasty had happened to me. My circumstances, however, were fine. I was healthy, intelligent and well-qualified. I had a good and interesting job, pleasant friends and a loving family in the south. So, what was going wrong? 'This is ridiculous,' I thought. 'I've done everything right, haven't I?' I wanted to beat my head against the wall, to smash it to pulp, to beat sense into my aberrant brain. How could I be so senseless yet so aware? I took long, brisk walks in terrible weather, trying to drive the infuriated agitation out of my body. I hadn't cried for a long time, so I wasn't getting any relief that way.

In desperation, I spoke to my manager at work. I had to apologise, to compensate for the awful dreadfulness of me. How had they ended up with me? I had innocently deceived them, presenting myself as a good, well-motivated, qualified employee. A safe bet. I told her I was overwhelmed and exhausted by the job and wanted to leave. She asked me about my future plans. I was caught off guard; this was not part of my script. I'd considered this conversation in advance, but it was a one-sided consideration. I'd planned to control the dialogue and not let the impetus pass to her, but there wasn't an answer to her question. What plans did I have other than not being here? I couldn't offer a satisfactory alternative life. What business of hers was it anyway? I was a grown up, not a vulnerable child running away from home, with savings and family, and I was unlikely to be taken advantage of, in a railway underpass, in return for a roof over my head.

'I think you should go and see your GP to discuss all this,' she said. 'I think this could be helped, perhaps with antidepressants. Lots of people take them, and you might find life easier.' I was startled. My fervent, and patently justifiable desire to guillotine my life was clearly seen as a welfare issue. Was I really doing such a bad job? If I had been, this would have been the perfect opportunity to let me go.

So, I thought: 'Oh well, I could give it a go,' though I wasn't clear how it was going to improve matters. I never saw doctors as, up to now, I had been an extremely healthy, lucky person. I'd last seen a GP, when unwell, as an eleven year old with an infected foot and had been prescribed surprising, bright red and black penicillin capsules. I'd thought I was swallowing plastic and, as I didn't share my anxiety, nobody had a chance to reassure me. A previous job had required me to have a private medical (so not at my registered GP's surgery), which I had easily passed, but remembered vividly and uncomfortably, as it seemed to involve a breast examination that took a very long time indeed. I had my doubts about that male doctor but, as I desperately wanted the job, I thought I'd better not complain. It was probably nothing anyway, just my imagination. However, doctors, in my eyes, were best avoided and although I'd lived in the town for nine months, I was still registered with a GP practice 200 miles away.

My GP selection process was as unsophisticated as usual. I didn't ask other people for a recommendation, which would have been sensible, I just wandered round the central area and chose the surgery building I liked best - elegant late Georgian this time. The receptionist was very unfriendly, until I realised I'd presented my NHS card with the incomprehensible foreign language side uppermost ... otherwise known as Welsh. I wasn't surprised it puzzled her. Welsh is a perfectly functional language, but a page of Welsh is alarmingly consonant rich to the uninitiated. After that, we got on quite well as I was clearly an inoffensive, British local. It was an interesting experience, as it made me realise that my self-assumed and rather dramatic or paranoid outsider status, largely a result of my southern accent, was nothing like the harsh realities of being a foreign immigrant.

I was offered a late afternoon appointment. It was August, and another sunny day, but I hadn't really noticed as I was highly anxious and uncomfortable. The GP was new to the practice. He was about my age and turned out to be very nice. I was well and considerately treated. We discussed the effects of stress and possible lifestyle changes; perhaps taking up a new hobby or sport. I was calm, rational and polite, but I wondered why we were having this conversation. I couldn't see that enrolling in an evening class was going to make things better. At the end, he told me, 'Come back if things don't improve.' I left, feeling vaguely as though we'd had a conversation about pets when I was actually planning a holiday to France.

'Well, that's that,' I thought. 'I was right all along; I'm not ill at all.' A bubble of excitement and relief filled my chest, and the air was suddenly thin and light. The golden early evening sunshine, that I'd barely noticed before, made the red brick buildings glow vibrantly crimson. This good feeling didn't last long, as I soon realised that, while it was nice to have been proved right, having an illness would have made everything so much easier. It would have been something else to blame, rather than just my normal self. I could, perhaps, have had some time away from work and a chance to mentally regroup, but, no, it was business as usual. The medical route had been explored and dismissed - if not exactly by the doctor, it had certainly been dismissed by me. I didn't plan to go back to see the GP again, as it would be wasting his time if I wasn't ill. Why should a GP have had to listen to me moaning about my life? He was a medical professional, not an agony aunt.

I reported back to my manager: 'There's nothing wrong. Everything's fine.' I should now be triumphant. I'd won the argument, hadn't I? This wasn't a welfare issue at all. She was surprised at the outcome. I suspect she thought I might have been less than truthful, but that wasn't exactly the issue. I was just too passive, too polite, and let the conversation follow the GP's expectations. He'd probably seen a slightly overstressed, middle class female working in the arts, likely neurotic, but they're all like that, aren't they? Nothing to worry about; she'd be back in due course, to whine about something or other else. Well, that's what I suspected he thought. As usual, I'd superimposed my beliefs about myself on someone else with precisely no evidence to support my particular hypothesis.

Now, I could walk away from this job. As an undeniably 'well person', my actions were perfectly justifiable and rational, but I'd lost the rash courage of a few weeks earlier. I'd been made to stop and think, and I soon realised that I hadn't really won the argument at all. I decided to stay a while and leave in a more considered fashion. It had taken a lot of effort to get this far and I was loath to throw everything away. It was definitely time to look at other jobs, although there were never many positions available in my area of work. I'd now been in my current job for nearly a year, just enough time for it to look fairly respectable on my CV. Hopefully, something could be salvaged from this bewildering, miserable experience.

Deep down though, for all my brave thoughts, I knew there was something very, very wrong. Time, in some unquantifiable way I couldn't quite specify, was running out. It was certainly getting to the stage that I hardly recognised myself. A year ago, I was happy and confident. I accompanied an exhibition (as a courier) to Japan, and then toured around Japan by myself. I was writing an essay for a London exhibition catalogue with a close, professional friend. Then I had, of course, decided it was time to apply for a new job with greater responsibility and higher pay. I knew I'd be a good candidate especially as I'd just passed my professional examinations; nobody would need to know my ingloriously low pass mark. That was me then. Normal.

And now what? I was spinning downwards, faster and faster. There's very little to say about this, as I really wasn't looking where I was going. There was absolutely no way I wanted to see, or think about, what might be at the bottom. Not at all.

Perhaps, it would have been better if I had looked, then maybe I could have pulled back before I reached madness. But when exactly was that? Could it have been timed? Was it the afternoon I'd skirted round the issue with the GP? Was there a precise moment when too much dopamine, or faulty mental wiring, or whatever it was, finally disrupted the usual operation of my brain?

I continued on with my daily life. I didn't know quite what else to do; it provided structure, if nothing else. At work, I remained a 'person of concern', but I don't remember being aware of this. Hence, the following recollections belong to my then manager. She recalls questioning my long, self-inflicted working hours. I, apparently, answered that I had to work long hours as I was 'inefficient'. This was, in fact, increasingly true. As I became more and more tired I was, inevitably, less and less productive. She also spoke to HR about me, but they weren't helpful, only suggesting that she should 'manage me better' and forbid me from overworking. Sadly, whatever my manager said to me, I don't think I took much notice. My overworking was an irrational, anxiety-driven compulsion and not amenable to reason. At this stage, I was fully aware this wasn't normal or healthy behaviour, but I didn't know how to rescue myself.

By now, I was sleeping less and less. I'd never had anything but transitory problems with sleep before but, by October, I had developed an unfamiliar sleep pattern with a forty eight hour cycle. One night my sleep was reasonable, the next non-existent. Insomnia was a new experience and it was baffling and frustrating. In my previous, easy world, sleep was just another function; it was another part of what the body did, rather like digestion or breathing. Not something you noticed, until it went wrong.

I discovered the barren hell of interminable sleepless nights, and how they ended with the cold, hard reality of getting up and starting all over again. I wasn't lying in bed worrying particularly, with a head full of anxious thoughts. It was more that I just *couldn't* sleep. I lived near the station, and for the first time I became obsessively aware of the train announcement system which started up at about 5.30 am. It was a virtual alarm clock because, of course, I was already awake. I went for long walks, avoided caffeine, and kept regular hours. Nothing helped.

Something, however, was changing and evolving in my brain. It was insidious. When did it happen the first time? The second time? The confirmatory third time? I don't know. My self-loathing and anger was reducing and there was a seismic shift in how I perceived myself. This should have been a good thing, but it wasn't because I was suddenly no longer alone. Instead, I now had an instant, unwanted, unpleasant special friend; a friend that nobody else saw or knew about. This friend was actually a strange arbitrary body of twelve ... erm ... somethings. I never quite found out who, or what, they were. They called themselves 'The Rules', so there was no doubt about their function. I wasn't at all happy about 'The Rules', particularly as they didn't seem to be any more enthusiastic about me than I currently was. In fact it was worse as, unfortunately, they seemed to be considerably more punitive and angry than me.

I didn't really question their existence; they just arrived one day, rather like a dodgy email. Where did they come from? I had absolutely no idea. Had anything like this happened to me before? Emphatically not. I passively accepted them, as if they were some form of unfortunate germ, like influenza, but I was rather ashamed of them, so I didn't discuss them with anyone else. After all, I'd presumably brought them on myself, as a punishment, but for what? Bad behaviour? It was mystifying. Surely, I hadn't behaved so badly that I'd been brought to the attention of a bunch of cosmic deliverers of justice? Or whatever they were. I had no idea what they looked like either. Who were these things, people, its? They were curiously one-dimensional, half-formed, but, nevertheless, they seemed to have compelling power.

I was now, most definitely, beginning to recalibrate my vision of myself. Yes, I was dreadful, but I was a victim too. I felt distinctly hard done by. 'Not fair, not fair,' yet again rattled around my head; the usual response of a naughty child thwarted by a, probably right, grown up.

About this time, a job came up not far away. It was a more junior job than my current one, but it was in a better institution. Promisingly, I already knew the person I would be assisting; as a student I'd done some voluntary work for one of her colleagues. So, I applied and, in due course, was invited for an interview. This was it, it was important. There weren't many sensible routes out of my current predicament, and there might not be another opportunity like this for quite some time. If I got the job I could commute while I sorted things out. The house purchase was still going through and I would probably withdraw from the transaction, but that was life, wasn't it?

I set off for the interview, nervously hopeful ... perhaps ... perhaps ... my life could be salvaged. But then 'The Rules' decided to interfere. My conversation with 'The Rules' went something like this:

Them: 'You were wrong to take the job you have already.'

Me: 'Erm, yes.'

Them: 'And now you're going to apply for another one. What makes you think you'll be any better this time round?'

Me: 'Well, umm ...'

Them: 'There's only one solution to this mess. You need to make sure that they know all your bad points in the interview so, if they really do decide to employ you, there will be no dishonesty involved.'

Me: 'Oh ... But I didn't lie on my CV, I never do.'

Them: 'We're not talking about your qualifications and experience, we're talking about your personal characteristics.'

Me: 'But I don't want to, that's not how interviews work. It'll look very peculiar. They won't give me the job.'

Them: 'You've got no choice. These are 'The Rules'.'

'These are 'The Rules' was soon to be a very familiar pronouncement, especially as there was never an alternative plan on offer. I dutifully spent a lot of time in the interview obsessively elucidating my bad points. The interview panel looked slightly confused and mildly fed up. Perhaps they thought I'd decided I didn't want the job anyway, and was deliberately wasting their time, but I did want that job. I wanted it so much. It was the only escape route on offer that could keep my life relatively intact.

The lead interviewer called me later, at home. Unsurprisingly, I wasn't successful. The job went to someone else, someone who was, no doubt, enthusiastic and confident during the interview. In fact, the way I'd normally behave in a job interview. A further comment was made: apparently I hadn't filled in the application form well; it was muddled, and they'd found it difficult to follow. I got the impression that they only interviewed me because I was already known to them. Either way, it was a nasty surprise as I had, over the years, produced innumerable pieces of carefully structured written work. Essay writing was at the core of my arts-based education. I knew all about job applications and usually went through the person specification meticulously, and then addressed it point by point. That's what I'd done this time, hadn't I?

I struggled onwards. I was tired and low, and now I'd got 'The Rules' to consider as well. It was overwhelming. At work, I packaged up some studio pottery to send back to its creator. I was fully aware I hadn't packed those pots well, but I was too tired and dispirited to look for more packaging and properly brace the sides of the boxes. The vases and bowls were damaged in transit and the potter was distraught. These were some of her favourite pieces.

I couldn't believe what I'd let myself do; it was totally out of character. I was used to being extremely careful when looking after ceramics. I was a museum curator, so I'd learnt how to store precious objects, how to handle them, how to display them and, most importantly of all, how not to damage them. What was happening to me? My known self seemed to be slipping away, and I desperately wanted to turn back the clock. How could I have caused this potter so much pain, simply because I couldn't be bothered? I asked her to provide a valuation of the damage, so we could process an insurance claim. It turned out to be about £600.

'The Rules' were not happy. To compensate, they announced that I should pay for the damage in person. So, I wrote a cheque on my current account and sent it to the potter. She was confused and rang me at work, a call I took while surrounded by my colleagues.

'I thought this was an insurance claim?' she asked, reasonably.

I muttered, 'Oh yes, it's just the way this is going to be done. Don't worry, just cash the cheque. It'll be sorted out later.'

She told me, again, that the money wasn't much of a compensation for the damage I'd done. I never knew if she cashed my cheque. I hope she did, but I didn't, and wouldn't, look. It was too painful and humiliating, and I only knew there was enough money in my account to pay her because I didn't spend all of my salary each month. Goodness knows what she made of this strange transaction. I had made the organisation I worked for look deeply unprofessional and was horribly embarrassed by the whole affair.

Were 'The Rules' happy? I'd done what they'd ordered, hadn't I? No, they were never happy. I was not thanked for following their instructions; this was apparently a time for punishment rather than congratulation.

Apart from this disastrous episode, I was actually doing OK at work, though not for much longer, and my gloomy self-assessments sound, in retrospect, somewhat hysterical. Throughout the autumn of 1999, I was busy re-displaying the costume galleries with celebratory costumes and accessories, a quiet nod to the upcoming millennium. This milestone date was not very celebratory as far as I was concerned, but such is life. I didn't avoid the bits I found challenging; I saw through a related school project, organised loans of some more up to date garments, and sorted out the advertising to the best of my ability.

It was a big job and everything had to be in place for the new year, so it wasn't a deadline I could ignore, however I was feeling. I thought the galleries looked lovely by the time I'd finished working on them, and was particularly grateful to Mary, an older volunteer. She was a retired seamstress and she patiently and conscientiously sewed stretchy fabric together, to mask the mannequins' more disturbingly humanoid features.

Meanwhile, 'The Rules' continued to meddle in my life; I still couldn't take annual leave, for one thing. This prohibition had, of course, been going on for months, long before 'The Rules' appeared. Previously, however, this lack of holiday had been (just about) my decision. Not any longer, not when annual leave would have been particularly useful. The house purchase was nearly completed, and I was going to need time off to deal with domestic practicalities. It was all very frustrating but there was nothing I could do about it.

I never thought to ask 'The Rules' the vital question: 'If I don't do what you say, what's the worst you can do? Really?' It wasn't so much that I was afraid of what 'The Rules' might do, it was just that disobeying them wasn't possible. It appeared to be a done deal; one I seemed to have magically signed up to while not paying attention. I wished that I hadn't entered into this curious arrangement but that was as far as it went. There didn't appear to be a get-out clause on offer, and I don't remember looking for one, as I somehow knew it would be pointless.

CHAPTER 4 MALIGNANT CONTROL

It was now December 1999, and my house purchase was finally complete. It had taken a long time and the poor sellers were not impressed. I had waited politely for my solicitors to process the paperwork, unaware that I was supposed to chivvy them along. When I finally realised this useful fact and made a nuisance of myself, it worked. I was, for the first time, a homeowner.

It was a good feeling; something else achieved in life, and security at last. No more landlords. The last landlord never refunded my deposit, although there was no reason for him to withhold it. He was full of slippery promises and, somehow, the money never quite materialised. The law hadn't changed yet to protect blameless tenants, and it was, at the time, a common complaint. It wasn't the first time it had happened to me. He was lucky; I didn't bother fighting for my money, as I was too hemmed in by my other problems.

My move was, at best, OK. Thanks to 'The Rules', I was permitted one weekday to move, and that was a concession because my removal men didn't work weekends. Luckily, even 'The Rules' hadn't insisted I buy a wheelbarrow and spend my evenings trundling my furniture through the town centre. As a result, there was no time to unpack anything; I was straight back to the office. A lot of my possessions were never rescued from their cardboard boxes until I moved again over two years later. It gave the house a shifty, unreliable look, as though I was permanently planning a midnight flit.

More fundamentally, I wasn't quite so sure about the house now anyway - my new exciting, much anticipated purchase. Yes, the square was beautiful, but the house, quite apart from the boxes, had a slightly evasive, treacherous feel to it. What the Germans call *unheimlich*. I wasn't sure why. The sellers seemed to have been decent enough. I didn't get surprise visits from alarming people or from bailiffs wanting to impound the television. There was a bit of damp but no vermin. Perhaps this unsettling feeling was nothing anyway as nowhere looks its best in damp, dark December. This was a new space for me to colonise, that was all. I knew it would be fine, once I'd added my character to it, and friends and family had come for the obligatory inspection. Why wouldn't it be? It was just a pile of ageing bricks and mortar, nothing more.

I hoped a few home improvements would help. The mortgage company required me to put in an attic wall, so that I didn't share my roof space with the house next door. As I had to employ a builder, I decided that this would be a good opportunity to reinstate the internal wall between the downstairs front and back room. The house felt spiritually fractured, with its face overlooking the benign, balanced, historic square, and its back overlooking wasteland and seething traffic. I needed to reconcile the two. Replacing the internal wall should help, I hoped, as it would create two, roughly cube shaped rooms - one for the back of the house, which I could then avoid, and one for the front, where I felt far safer. The cube-shaped room is one of the harmonic laws of classical architecture, both aesthetically pleasing and spiritually complete. I hoped it would bring some solidity to my untrustworthy house.

Then there were the watchers. Real or not real? It certainly made no sense. When I was in the front room, at night, with my back to the rear window, it felt as though I was being watched from behind. This was impossible. The rear window overlooked a small, high walled yard with an internally bolted gate. Beyond, there was nothing but the rough wasteland and a major road. Was it something to do with the wasteland? What had been there previously? It had the forlorn, coarse lumpiness of demolished buildings. Was there some kind of negative energy floating about, homeless after the demolitions? Surely, nobody could possibly be camping in my cold and bare backyard and, more to the point, why would they want to? Perhaps it was no more than a draught. That would explain the gentle, but icy, breath on my prickling neck, but not the uneasy feeling in my stomach.

I decided to get the building work done as soon as possible, so I could be physically separated from that worrying, rear window. Fortunately, there was some good news from 'The Rules'. Annual leave was allowed again ... provided I didn't take too much. Just in case. It was not so much that I was permitted to take leave, but rather that they didn't notice if I did.'Perhaps they're busy elsewhere,' I thought, keeping my head down. I bought a cooker and had it installed, got the phone line reconnected and worked through other minor domestic necessities.

My sleep was getting gradually worse. I would have given anything to have the forty eight hour cycle again. Now, I hardly slept at all. I was all too aware of my insomnia because my new house overlooked a church, and its clock struck every single hour. My hazy, wearisome, interminable nights were now actively alarming me. I panicked that I couldn't remember things: my postcode, my pin number, my phone number. I had never had a problem like this before. I'd believed that remembering these things was inbuilt, but I was now discovering that they were not; it was some kind of executive function that I was losing. A sort of early dementia? When was this going to stop? What else was I going to forget? I recalled an Enid Blyton cautionary tale from my childhood, a tale of a little girl who couldn't be bothered to remember things, so lost part of her brain in the woods. It was a sort of juvenile horror story, although all she missed were exciting events like parties and the circus. I wasn't too worried about parties and circuses, but I was very perturbed, and not all clear, about the whereabouts of a very useful part of my brain.

Worst of all, reality was beginning to shift again. Perhaps this explained the recent relative benevolence of 'The Rules'. I wasn't clear whether they were gradually revealing more of themselves and reforming, or whether there were totally new dictators in my life, and 'The Rules' had simply departed, in the rather inexplicable way they'd arrived.

Instead, there were goblins.

Yes, goblins. Not fairies, or elves, or pixies ... These entities wished to be known, and recognised, as goblins. Whether I was aware of it or not, it looks as though the goblins were an evolution of 'The Rules'; a sort of bolted on extra layer.

But goblins, I mean, seriously? It must be a bad joke. Who on earth believes in goblins? People just don't, and I most certainly didn't. I hadn't given them a thought since childhood.

I dimly remembered that they weren't very nice, and generally caused mayhem in Toyland - back to Enid Blyton. I obviously needed a protective Big Ears. But he was a gnome, wasn't he? Gnomes don't exist. Or unicorns, or water sprites, or Tinkerbell. I wasn't even convinced about God. I would have described myself as agnostic; I wasn't a full out atheist because all those Christians could well be right. I vaguely understood faith as a gift of God, but I always believed I had the wrong kind of brain for faith; I was too prosaic.

Now, I seemed to have discovered a faith of sorts. I wished it was faith in something positive and culturally acceptable – well, God really would have been a good start. My family and friends would have been surprised, but as long as I was happy they wouldn't worry. I could have gone to the church across the street and mixed with like-minded people, enjoying the reassuring community of belief. I could have taken up good works, and become a valuable contributor to society. But, as luck would have it, I seemed to have got the wrong kind of faith. It was certainly not God. There was no obvious community of like-minded people I could join and, before easy internet access, I couldn't go searching for fellow believers across the world.

I appeared to be totally alone with my fairyland squatters. They had set up their home in my home, especially favouring those cracks in the old plaster that the surveyor had assured me were structurally insignificant and basically harmless. That much was true but it appeared, instead, that these cracks were psychically, hugely important. Perhaps these new goblins were the downstairs watchers too. Itchy, witchy, scratchy, tiny goblins. They chittered and chattered, mostly after dark. They were unpleasant and seedy but ridiculous, obviously. I could feel laughter squirming and curling up from my stomach. It was painful; look the other way, and laugh. However, laughing at goblins turned out to be a big mistake. The more I tried to diminish and dismiss them, the more insistent they became. I was being coerced into new beliefs, and they were not helpful in the least.

The New Year was particularly memorable for me and that wasn't only because it was the millennium. Parties, fireworks and, in this northerly part of the country, pouring rain at midnight. The millennium bug came to nothing, and the doomsayers and soothsayers had to face up to life as normal. There was no appreciable distinction between 31st December 1999 and 1st of January 2000, except the weather was better. Practically speaking, they felt the same.

I spent the 31st at my manager's house with her family; her middle class road, in a neighbouring town, had its own millennium street party. She was reaching out to me because she was still concerned - 'fragile' is how she describes it now. Fragile? I guess she was right, at least mentally speaking, but it's not a description I'd have chosen for myself at the time. She was a kind lady. I wasn't a good or considerate guest as, at some point during the evening, feeling exhausted and pressured, I drifted off into the rain-washed surrounding streets. To my horror, my absence was noticed, and my manager drove round in her car until she found me. I'm embarrassed about that, even now.

In my defence, I was coming to the end of my tether. I couldn't face any more sleepless nights and the, so called, amusing goblins, were not being amusing in the least. They were beginning to manifest themselves in other ways. The plaster-dwelling goblins were very small, but these new goblins were much larger, about eighteen inches high. They were greenish brown, wizened, twiggy little old men - like a drawing by Arthur Rackham, whose illustrations I'd always admired. When making pronouncements, of the type previously issued by 'The Rules', twelve of them would come together, forming a sort of council and tidily aligning themselves in two rows of six. These larger goblins also preferred the hours of darkness. During the long winter evenings they drifted around the house, usually when my back was turned, and congregated in corners, particularly in the rather forlorn kitchen. They also infested the tiny front garden and were, I suspected, spreading throughout the neighbourhood, taking up residence in all sorts of random greenery outside. It was becoming increasingly difficult to evade them, at least at home. Had the goblins infiltrated my workplace yet? I can't remember. Either way, I seemed to be increasingly watched and increasingly monitored. It was all very unsettling and I was deeply confused. Why did these strange beings find me so interesting?

By January, I was totally shattered - house moving; 'The Rules', followed by goblins; the big millennium exhibition at work; and, most of all, my continuing insomnia, had wiped me out. One evening, shortly after the New Year, I remember having a bath and reflecting gloomily on my situation. I really didn't know what to do. It didn't occur to me that I might be ill. After all goblins were the stuff of nightmares, not disease, and nightmares were ephemeral, not real. You would reassure a nightmare ridden child, and the child was supposed to take comfort, face up to the monster, and move on, a braver and happier, little person. If I admitted to anyone what had been happening, I expected the same would happen to me. I would be reassured by kind people, laughed at by less kind people and, overall, be expected to overcome my fears.

This scenario was both depressing and embarrassing. If I could defeat my fears, surely I would have done it by now? I was obviously, as usual, not being strong minded enough. I seemed to have regressed and got stuck in the worst part of someone else's horrible childhood. Yes, I had been a nervous child, frightened by all sorts of things, but those anxieties had hardly defined my life. Overall, I had been reasonably well adjusted and my school career had been unremarkable. My autobiographical memories were predominantly happy, and I didn't remember anything more than the usual life traumas.

Now, things were different. I really needed to discuss matters with someone. I'd had months of keeping these peculiar problems to myself, and they just seemed to be getting worse and worse. I didn't feel able to speak to my family. I'm not sure what they could have added, as I had already applied my family's values to the problem. These were broadly my values, the values I was brought up with, and they hadn't really solved anything so far. I imagined my family hurt, upset, worried, and unable to help and then, rather less nobly, having a good laugh at the idea of goblins. Black comedy was used as a defensive mechanism in our family, a panacea when faced with disaster, and it did nothing for my pride. I wanted to keep up appearances. I was a successful daughter living independently, with a good job and loving my new house. There were also younger siblings still living at home and the focus should be on them, not me. I was already successfully launched, so to speak.

Or so I'd thought. My adult life felt increasingly impossible. However, as I wasn't ill, there would be no opportunity to have a recuperative break. As work was a pressing concern, I decided, somewhat bleakly, I'd better speak to my manager as a sort of follow up to the summer 'welfare' conversation. Let her know what was going on, and why I seemed to be even more hopeless than usual.

The goblins, who were hanging about in the bathroom (I never got any privacy, but I just accepted that as another done deal), were quiet during this internal bath time soliloquy, but once they realised I intended to go public, they were suddenly agitated and announced:

'If you tell anyone they will betray you. You are not allowed to speak of us.' They used their usual creaky, nasty old men voices, which were never very expressive, but their word choice was deeply emotive. 'Not allowed,' I understood well enough, as I'd had plenty of random diktats prefaced with that over the last few months, but 'betray?' How had betrayal suddenly become part of the conversation?

I was deeply, deeply scared. My relationship with these strange beings was sinisterly evolving. The use of the word 'betray' was less of a warning; it was more of a threat. This was the first time I'd felt so overtly threatened. It was not an Archimedes moment. Instead of leaping out of the bath, enjoying a burst of enlightenment, I sat and shivered in the increasingly tepid bathwater, suddenly totally lost in time and space. I'd got used to going along with all sorts of unhelpful behaviour, but that's because I believed I ultimately didn't have an option. There had been no reason to threaten me before, as I'd been generally obedient. But not now. This response was so frightening, that I was determined to bring the goblins into the metaphorical open air. They'd spent enough time festering, more or less quietly, in my closed-up world. It wasn't going to be an easy conversation. I was sick with dread, and was desperate to get it over and done with, but I had to wait for my manager to come back from leave.

Our conversation was, predictably, uncomfortable for both of us. I went through the usual sad litany of the maladjusted employee: 'I can't concentrate, I can't sleep, I can't do my job ...' and then, deep breath, the sucker punch. 'And I'm being told what to do by goblins.'

There was a very long silence indeed. I'd managed to take the conversation from the drearily predictable to the completely bizarre, in one sentence. My manager was no doubt mentally flicking through the *How to be a Good Manager* handbook, looking for the section entitled 'Totally bananas ...' Not that I saw it that way. 'Bananas', however it was defined, was well down my list of possible explanations, but I wasn't so far from reality there wasn't a small part of me thinking: 'This is all very strange ... and I'm not sure it's quite as supernatural as I think,' or was being made to think. But that was a small fugitive part and it was, of necessity, well concealed from bossy goblins.

My manager prevaricated a bit, and said she needed to think about what I had just told her. After all, what do you say to someone like me? Effectively, she meant she was going to take further advice, but I didn't realise this and was somewhat mystified by the delay. The following day I was told that I must make an appointment with my GP, and tell him everything I had told her and most especially the bit about the goblins. I must also take a week's holiday. At least, thanks to 'The Rules', I had a lot of annual leave left, so that wasn't a problem.

I spent part of the week stripping wallpaper in the front room. The goblins had no views about this, so it was a cathartic activity that didn't require any brain power. Which was just as well, as I hadn't got any. At some point, I lined the walls and painted the room green. The goblins were happy with this choice but, even without their input, green was (and is) my favourite colour, so it was a conflict-free decision. The room looked lovely, but it was just as well that I had no idea that this would be the first and last room I would decorate in my much anticipated new home.

The hall and landing were more problematic, as they'd been thoroughly coated in a hard, swirling plaster and painted white. It would have been sensible to employ a plasterer to cover this up, or learn to live with it. After all, it was only the hall, not a living space. The goblins, however, were extremely keen to see it removed, possibly so they could infest the softer, more friable plaster behind. There again, perhaps it was no more than a random, goblin punishment. As usual, there was little rhyme or reason to them. Why the hall plaster was so interesting to them and the front room wallpaper wasn't, was beyond me. None of my business, probably.

I dejectedly chipped away at the hall for ages. It must have driven my poor neighbour mad, because my hall was next to his front room, and my landing was next to his front bedroom.

It was dusty, dirty hard work and I really didn't want to do it. Getting at the top of the walls was impossible, as the house had high ceilings, so it was a pretty pointless, unrewarding activity. The hall ended up with a strange, ragged skirt of unremoved plaster, which was still there when I moved, over two years later. It was annoying; there were so many more rewarding projects that I wanted to get done in my new home.

At least, when not decorating, I enjoyed lots of fresh air. This was obviously a good thing, although it wasn't quite in the manner I would have chosen for myself. The goblins ordered me to take long walks but, for some reason never divulged, they favoured the middle of the night. This was January, when it was not only dangerous, but very cold. They had me roaming around deserted streets in some of the better areas; they admired the trees there, which were admittedly pretty impressive under the orange streetlights. Not that you'd find a goblin in a large tree; they preferred to lurk in bushes. The town was very quiet and I didn't come to any harm, but I would have preferred my rambles to have been during daylight hours.

As for the GP appointment? It had to wait. My GP, it appeared, had just gone on holiday. 'Is it urgent?' the receptionist asked. I considered heart attacks, pneumonia and other life threatening conditions. I appeared to have a psychic infection, but you could hardly treat that with antibiotics, so I said 'No,' and was offered a routine appointment in two and half weeks' time.

After my compulsory week off, I went back to work. What was I working on after the New Year? I don't remember, but I was lucky. With a big exhibition recently completed, I could keep my increasingly distracted head down. I suspect I was mostly busy with low level housekeeping, including the horribly stressful job - ceramics were the worst - of cleaning the display cases in the galleries, which seemed to grow their own dust. At least I was now working in a relatively small gallery and museum. My previous job had required a lot of dusting, not just the display cases but also the seemingly innumerable sculptures that garnished that splendid building. I would wander round for hours, with my stepladder, small brush and cylindrical vacuum cleaner, wondering why I wasn't allowed to use a duster and, more profoundly, why I'd thought becoming a museum curator was a good idea in the first place - particularly as I edged along stone ledges, with sheer drops to the stone staircases below. Luckily, I wasn't afraid of heights. But who was it who drew pencil rings around the chaste nipples of naked, marble ladies? Such tiny, anarchic moments. Disaffected teenagers, bored on school trips? Why, just why?

Meanwhile, back in the present, my poor manager was increasingly agitated.

'Have you seen your GP yet?' she kept asking. 'If you don't go soon, I'll march you down there myself!'

To which my answer was: 'He's on holiday, I've got an appointment when returns.' While thinking, 'for goodness sake get off my back, I can't drag him back from whatever he's doing.' Skiing, I speculated, as it was January and he looked sporty, but I'd absolutely no idea really.

I wasn't sure why she was so anxious; I had no empathy for her state of mind in the least. Looking back, I suspect I was now a profoundly worrying member of staff, but I didn't understand this at all, so saw no reason to speed things along. After all, my unhappy situation had been more or less like this for weeks, and how much did I really want to chat to the GP anyway? The goblins were, unsurprisingly, extremely unhappy about that particular suggestion. Was it worth upsetting them to such an extent? Could anyone really fix what was going on, or was I basically buggered?

I wasn't entirely sure that my soul was totally mine anymore, but this was a rather puzzling consideration. How had I managed to compromise it? Was this some kind of religious or story book scenario, where I'd entered into a contract with the Devil? Perhaps the goblins were representatives of the Devil? But surely, if I'd entered into a contract, I'd get something out of it? Being told what to do was a poor reward, as far as I was concerned. I was very used to being independent and I certainly wasn't looking for any directions from outsiders - at least not consciously. If I was looking for external support, unpleasant goblins wouldn't have been at the top of my list, or anybody else's, for that matter.

CHAPTER 5 MEDICAL MATTERS

For the first time, everything I say to people is going to be documented. It's probably just as well that at the time I didn't know this was going to happen, and that my problems with goblins were about to become public - to a whole range of mental health professionals.

I've been an unreliable narrator so far, as I've been the sole reporter of this case. Now, there are medical notes from 2000-2002; a lot of medical notes. I have copies of everything, including the separate notes that were kept by the community mental health team. At that time, patients didn't receive copies of clinic letters so, unless you specifically requested to see them, you had no idea of what was written about you. I paid for copies of my medical notes some years after I left the town, and they were very painful reading but incredibly helpful. For the first time I considered other people's perspective of my illness, and not just my own. How different these perspectives were: what I interpreted as coercion and interference, was mostly the result of completely unappreciated attempts to help me. A lot of time and effort went into this, and most of it was pretty fruitless as I had no idea that people were trying their best for me.

I will use these to help reconstruct what happened, as my memory - apart from certain salient events - is increasingly hazy and unreliable, although I usually do have a clear recollection of how I felt. The notes give my story a coherent structure I can't provide otherwise, and they also provide quite a lot of details about what I believed. I can outline a broad framework, but it's without the details and, especially, the dates.

The GP appointment came round eventually. It was early evening and, unlike the warm sunny August of the last appointment, it was now cold and dark. The surgery was busy and we, the patients, waited on grey, foam covered benches. The building might be elegant but the waiting room furniture was not.

I waited, feeling sick. Announcing to anyone, 'I'm being told what to do by goblins,' was not something to look forward to. Would the GP accuse me of wasting his time? Or suggest that I just needed to grow up a bit and not indulge in nightmares? He was a nice man; it was more likely he'd be kind and, oh so slightly, disappointed. I'd had all that good advice in August, and had I followed any of it? No. Here I was, back again. 'Oh doctor. I can't cope, fix my life ...' I felt ashamed and apologetic.

Thankfully, the GP didn't ask me how much of his previous good advice I'd actually bothered to follow. This was a relief. I twisted the strap on my shoulder bag and stared at the floor, as he asked me what seemed to be a lot of rather difficult questions. It was hard work trying to remember and explain what had been going on, and it was a long and, to me, rather peculiar consultation. Why did he want to know all this stuff? I glanced at my watch and felt guilty about all those people in the waiting room. What could they be thinking I was doing? They'd have seen me go in, as the consulting room door was visible from the waiting room.

I prepared myself for the GP's summing up, along the lines of, 'I don't think there's anything to worry about.' One side of me wanted to hear that; it meant I could pull myself together and engage properly with life. Well, that was the theory, but I wasn't doing too well so far. The other, more realistic side, was dubious that it would really be a useful response. As I was totally unprepared for the verdict, it came as a shock. 'I'm going to refer you to a psychiatrist,' he said. 'You shouldn't have to wait long. Don't worry; she's very nice.' He also prescribed sleeping tablets. I took one, slept better, then, the following day, nearly got run over crossing a dual carriageway on my walk to work. So, I put them to one side, thinking, 'I'm not sure that was a great idea.'

What was going on? Why did I need to see a psychiatrist? I didn't ask the doctor why he thought this was a good idea, as I was pretty well stunned into silence. The impact of my statements totally passed me by: I was a well-educated, thirty one year old with a responsible job, who had apparently abandoned her usual, unexceptionable and unexceptional place in life, in favour of deferring to some small, greenish brown, unpleasant creatures usually found in fairy tales. As you do. Or rather, as you don't. That was the problem.

I'd met a psychiatrist once before, when I was eighteen and about to drop out of university. There's very little of that encounter that stays with me. I remember being asked about birth trauma - which I found mystifying. Surely, he'd be better off asking my mother if she'd found my birth traumatic; all I'd been told was that it was a very wet year and there was a plague of daddy-long-legs. This story was regularly aired every time someone at home came across a limp, hopeless daddy-long-legs, drippily lurking in a ceiling corner over the lavatory and therefore, insultingly, analogous to me - a comment on my character, not my appearance. Ho ho ho; sometimes family jokes are painfully prescient.

Even I could see that this wasn't really what the psychiatrist was after. Then he wanted to know whether I thought people were talking about me. He was very insistent on that point. The answer to that was, 'I don't'. It was a baffling question. Why would people be talking about me? I didn't think I was especially boring, I certainly wasn't given to hanging around train stations with a notebook and a packed lunch, but neither did I consider myself especially interesting either. That had been that. I'd not attended the follow up and, after a few months, got on with life. Case closed, although the episode was somewhat troubling, and it was something I'd worked hard to forget, though I did, unwillingly, include my abortive university experience in my CV.

There was a happy ending anyway. I worked for a while, then enrolled in another university a couple of years later, had a fantastic time and got a good degree. Coincidentally, it was that degree that had led to another encounter with mental health services - just enough to frighten me - but this time I was, thankfully, not a patient.

I'd researched a local furniture retailer and manufacturer for my final year university dissertation. Local archives turned up a rich, previously unexplored, history of furnishing late nineteenth and early twentieth century public buildings. I assiduously visited as many as I could identify, rattling round the area on cheap day bus tickets, taking bad photographs in the low winter light. It was before the age of camera phones and I found 'real' cameras challenging. Rochdale bus station (on my way to Nelson, which appeared to be the end of the line in more ways than one) was especially memorable as it had its own resident flasher. Ah, Rochdale - Gracie Fields, the birth of the co-operative movement and well, erm ... I haven't been back.

Mayors' Parlours, found in the proudly built, nineteenth century town halls of the northern, industrial towns, were very rewarding as they were stuffed full of their original sturdy furniture. However, NHS and other healthcare buildings were far less fruitful, especially as many institutions had reinvented themselves several times - modern hospitals tend not to be so literally described as the 'St Catherine's Home for Inebriate Women'. Pre-internet, they could also be difficult to locate. However, I was more hopeful when it came to the old lunatic asylums - they might have dropped the word 'pauper' from their official names, but they were still, in the early 1990s, just about functioning as hospitals.

I remember visiting Stanley Royd, which had its own museum, a sort of random assemblage of psychiatric odds and ends. (This museum still exists at another location). In those days, I doubt it received many visitors, and the (honorary?) curator greeted me enthusiastically, keen to show off his star exhibits. He was particularly proud of the padded cell; a rare survivor (unsurprisingly) which, I think, may have been rented out to film companies. I can't imagine why anyone else would want to rent a padded cell unless they were having a very melodramatic Halloween party, and Halloween was rather less celebrated in the early 1990s. It looked horrible. I had expected it to see a clinical, shiny, white cell, but instead it seemed to be lined with the kind of grubby, whitish vinyl more often found on fly-tipped headboards. He then threw open the doors of a cupboard and produced a very mundane, medium sized, metal bucket. I gazed at it warily. Now what? I soon learnt. A poor lost soul had managed to drown themselves in it. Oh God. What desperation, what resolution. How many other horrors could this curator produce?

I'll never know, as by this stage I was desperately trying to inspect some utilitarian pieces of furniture, not esoteric in the least, of the type supplied to the matron's sitting room. Perhaps these would bear the paper label of the furniture firm I was researching. The curator seemed distinctly puzzled and was almost actively unhelpful. I suspect it was the first and last time he'd been visited by someone so passionately interested in a small, plain, light oak bookcase, and so unenthusiastic when it came to his more gruesome exhibits. I can't remember whether I found any relevant furniture as, unsurprisingly, the visit was unforgettable for other reasons.

Then there was High Royds, which was magnificently, gothically sinister in the best Hammer House of Horror way: a place of long, oppressively crypt-like corridors, with the ones nearest the main entrance ornately decorated with greenish mustard-colour tiles under grandly-patterned ceilings. Most of the hospital was now deserted, although I glimpsed a few patients behind locked wooden doors in the stairwells. 'We don't want to go that way,' a nice (if somewhat baffled by my interest in dull furniture) lady said. 'They use those stairs as toilets.' Did she really say that? Those last, semi-visible patients were long term residents with learning disabilities. The idea that they were so uncared for that nobody bothered to ensure they used lavatories was deeply disturbing. How little respect was given to those abandoned wrecks of humanity.

My guide showed me some old furniture, brought together in

an enormous empty ward that was rather like a deserted factory building, but this furniture was labelled by a contemporary competitor of my firm. I left; it had been a pointless trip, and walked out into the raw, dripping afternoon of slowly thawing snow, consciously glad that I had the freedom to leave. The front lawns were fenced in by dense, soggy black trees. It was uncannily quiet away from the city and, as I walked away, I could feel the enormous bulk of the building, alive, its every blank window watching me from behind. Who knew what strange, disturbing thoughts and emotions were trapped in those old buildings? Who had looked out of those windows? Why were they there? What had they done? Although it was a shadowless day, deeply overcast and not far from dusk, I felt the long finger of the clock tower icily marking my back. Perhaps, that was the day I contracted madness - as yet a dormant madness, lurking in an unregarded part of my brain.

After graduation, I'd busily moved on with life and started on the museum career path that had led me here. The troubled eighteen year old had been banished for good, I believed, feeling very pleased with myself. Pride goes before a fall. It was likely that proud self- sufficiency which so annoyed the furious poet.

And now? I had an appointment to see a psychiatrist at the local hospital. I had no idea what this hospital looked like, but I knew that it was not the old, enormous lunatic asylum on the fringes of the town, that was now mostly unused. This, I guess, was faintly reassuring, but overall this appointment was, most definitely, not in my life script. As I was entirely unaware of how NHS waiting times work, I didn't realise my referral was urgent. It was a weekday afternoon, cold and grey but otherwise nondescript; the hospital was about an hour's walk from home. The psychiatric unit turned out to be in a secluded area towards the back of the hospital, along with hearing aids and sexual health. I wondered how the deaf old ladies felt, sandwiched between the loonies (me) and those whose morals were 'probably not all that they should be' (not me, chance would be a fine thing).

I expected the waiting room to be busy, but it was eerily quiet. Where was everyone? There were only two people there, a receptionist/administrator in a plastic enclosed booth, and a very strange, young man. He paced around muttering to himself, then stretched himself full length on the waiting room furniture, and then, repetitively and forcefully, told the receptionist that he needed to see someone 'NOW!' She, solidly and persistently, told him that he saw someone only yesterday. The argument went round in circles, while I sat gazing at the floor, disquieted by this glimpse of an entirely new world, a world I really didn't want to enter at all. Now was not the time for accidental eye contact. I covertly inspected the waiting room furniture, which appeared to have escaped from a Burt Reynolds film, circa 1973. It was made up of hexagonal, free standing couches upholstered in a jolly, orange plastic. I had never seen anything quite like it in real life, and I'd lived through the seventies.

I waited, feeling sick again. Announcing to anyone, 'I'm being told what to do by goblins,' was not something to look forward to. There was a definite feeling of deja vu here.

I was called in. It was time for the goblins again. Great. There was not much to say about the first part of the interview. The psychiatrist, I'll call her Dr R, was pleasant and thorough.

We went through my mostly uneventful life in what felt like forensic detail and I carefully explained my countless character failings. Now was not the time to enumerate my good points, I concluded; that wasn't why I was here. However, I assured her correctly that I rarely drank, had never smoked or taken illegal drugs, or abused legal drugs such as pain killers.

Dr R then asked numerous questions about the goblins, 'The Rules' and all the rest. It felt like an educational, oral examination, so I diligently applied myself to the questions. Dr R clearly wished me, I decided, to discriminate between real and not real, and to think logically about my experiences. As required, I disengaged from my story and tried to regard it dispassionately, as a sort of intellectual conundrum. I said quite a lot of correct things on the subject but I didn't believe them, and it felt as though we were at cross-purposes. Why were we playing abstract games anyway? That wouldn't solve anything, would it? I'd still be stuck with the goblins. I was horribly conflicted and frustrated. Why didn't Dr R understand about the goblins and how they worked? What was the problem here? It was all straightforward, surely? Why didn't she get what I was saying? I was being perfectly clear, wasn't I? In my eyes, understanding the goblin modus operandi was no more complex than, say, painting a wall. If this had been a real oral exam, I would have failed. Big time.

Dr R also seemed to be disproportionately interested in what the goblins, and 'The Rules', had made me do. I didn't understand why this was so important to her, and I was very uncomfortable. I tried to explain that I didn't want to do the things required of me; it was just that I didn't have an option. I wasn't proud or glad about this, in fact it was something I was very unhappy about. If I wavered there were additional threats, for example they had threatened to destroy what was left of my concentration. How could I manage without any concentration whatsoever? I'd be reduced to the intellectual level of moss, and it would be goodbye to my treasured independence. But I couldn't actually do anything about it; it was just something I had to put up with and so, by implication, should she.

Finally, it was time for the verdict. Dr R told me my GP had thought me depressed but she didn't think I was. This was surprising; I felt depressed. Why wouldn't anyone be in my situation? (She did prescribe an antidepressant shortly afterwards, but, as I didn't seem to get any benefit, it was discontinued a few weeks later.) I was asked what I thought about medication in general. This question was a total and nasty surprise. Medication? Was I really ill? Wasn't I just trapped in some kind of childish nightmare, and needed to master whatever it was that was lurking under the bed? (Literally and metaphorically.) 'Oh yes, that's fine,' I lied politely, still the 'anxious to please' examination candidate. Inside, I was thinking, 'Oh dear God, help!' I hadn't learnt yet that psychiatrists tend to take everything at face value. It goes with the territory when recording the weird.

That was the appointment from my perspective, but now we have someone's else's point of view. This is taken from Dr R's letter to my GP, part of a much longer summary in my medical notes:

> *She gave an account of her symptoms in an extremely detached, unemotional way. Towards the end of the interview I did feel there was some rapport, and a little warmth, though she still had a most business-like manner when we discussed diagnosis and treatment. It was difficult to follow Jane's descriptions of her experiences with "the rules" as she took no account at all of what I might be likely to make of what she was saying, and I feel for someone of her obvious intelligence, this probably indicates some degree of thought disorder ...*
>
> *I think Jane clearly has a psychotic illness, but I am unclear as to its exact nature ...*
>
> *She herself thinks this may be depression ... however she does not seem to describe a degree of depression commensurate with a psychosis of this nature. In addition her delusions seem very bizarre. I think she may have some thought disorder and blunting of affect, and I note the long history of social withdrawal predating her symptoms ...*
>
> *I did not feel there was a significant risk of Jane harming herself or others although clearly this is a serious illness in which I have only a limited acquaintance with Jane, on her own account of the situation ...*

So, that's what it looked like from the outside. Business-like? Oh how un-business-like it felt. I was also 'extremely articulate' and was using a sort of DIY cognitive behavioural therapy. I should be proud of these comments, along with Dr R noting my intelligence. But I'm not, as they are rather embarrassing. I'm all too aware, with hindsight, that I soon will not be intelligent or articulate in the least and definitely not capable of DIY CBT.

I didn't realise, until I read these notes, that my mid-interview attempt at rapport had been totally misunderstood. I'd actually made a tiny little joke, referring to the slang term for Swiss bankers, 'The Gnomes of Zurich.' I can see now why this wouldn't have worked, but at the time it didn't occur to me that the psychiatrist wouldn't be able to differentiate between 'goblins' who were frightening and real, and 'gnomes' who were not frightening at all and definitely not real. As a result of her interview with me, people were always referring to my 'gnomes' rather than my 'goblins'. This would infuriate me, as the two were totally different, weren't they? How dare they insult the goblins by confusing them with benign, grandfatherly creatures who hung round garden ponds with fishing rods. Moral of this story: never make a flippant side remark to a psychiatrist, you'll find it recorded in your notes as fact. Just stick to the truth, however you want to define it.

I was given a prescription for an antipsychotic (sulpiride), a very general A4 information sheet about why I'd been prescribed one, and a blood test form. I was told about the day hospital, but I didn't like the sound of that at all, especially as it had the word 'hospital' in the description. 'No thank you; I've got a job to go to during the day,' turned out to be an acceptable response. A community psychiatric nurse would also be ringing me up. A community psychiatric who? Why on earth did I need one of those? Whatever they were.

I envisaged a Nurse Gladys type from *Open All Hours* sitting on my beat-up gallery sofa in my bare front room, and argued that I didn't think it was a good idea. I had enough trouble with unwanted goblins in my house, without having to cope with unknown, unwanted nurses as well. This, however, was not an acceptable response. I would be contacted by the nurse whether I liked it or not. I was beginning to suspect, entirely correctly, that psychiatrists, however pleasantly they present themselves, are actually, of necessity I suppose, rather bossy.

I took the blood test form round to phlebotomy and considered it while I was waiting.

'First episode psychosis'. I didn't know quite what this term meant, but I knew enough to realise that it was probably something I really didn't want. I was, apparently, officially ill, but I didn't feel ill, only tired and desperate. Everything in my life was going to have to be recalibrated. 'Oh dear,' I thought, 'none of this looks good, not good at all.' It had been an awful, bewildering afternoon.

Back at home, I thought with some relief that the dreadful day was now concluded, but I was wrong. The phone rang and it turned out to be the threatened psychiatric nurse. This nurse didn't sound like Nurse Gladys in the least. It was a deep-voiced man for starters. I told him why I really didn't want or need to see him. It was tricky for him as he was following instructions from Dr R, and I didn't understand medical hierarchies. However, he didn't insist. When he put down the phone I was shaking. I crouched on the floor and beat my head with my hands. I didn't want anybody else in my life; it was all too much. Goblins and now mental health services too. The goblins hung about in the corners of the room watching me. Unusually, they hadn't anything particular to say, but I knew what they were thinking. 'Serves you right .... we did try to warn you, and you wouldn't listen.' They were probably correct. What had I done?

CHAPTER 6 A LITTLE LEARNING

I was, at first, quite glad to have the antipsychotic medication, as I got to sleep properly for the first time in months. The 'not Gladys' psychiatric nurse (I'll now call him Sean, though it's not his real name) rang again and, this time, he came and visited too. He was a few years older than me and, to my startled surprise, extremely good looking in a, sort of, rough around the edges, George Clooney, way. But that, of course, was a peripheral observation, as he'd hardly come round to add a bit of Hollywood glamour to my dispiriting life. While I had no idea what Sean was like in his own home, he was, though I didn't yet know it, about to prove himself remarkably amiable and patient in his dealings with me.

As I was sleeping more, I felt more able to cope with things generally, and I reported back to both Sean and Dr R that the goblins had reduced their activities. My medical notes were quite upbeat but, for all this cautious optimism, my delusions seemed pretty secure. Yes, of course things improved, yet I was still standing on shifting sand. How much better were things really? How much did I just want them to be better and so squashed down all the uncomfortable, disquieting stuff, hoping it would, in some way, dissolve? This was how I normally dealt with the inconvenient bits of reality, so it was hardly surprising that it was my strategy of choice.

To be honest, I hadn't yet mastered the tricky business of being a patient, whereby being truthful is a necessity for a proper, trusting relationship. I politely lied to both the nurse and the psychiatrist because that's what you do in normal social discourse.

'How are you?' they'd ask.

'Fine, thanks,' I'd reply, and all the rest.

They wanted me to recover, I wanted to recover; so it was a satisfying answer for all of us. It also gave me access to the magical equation: 'If I tell you I'm well, you believe I'm well, so you tell me I'm well and therefore ... I AM WELL.' Bingo! This was a problem. As far as I was concerned, the existence of my illness - whatever I was told - was more subjective than objective, and if you really want to get better, accepting you are ill in the first place does make things easier.

I was also still struggling to explain the exact nature of the goblins to, well, everybody who asked. There are traces of my lack of true auditory and visual hallucinations throughout my medical notes, to the point where I actually gave up trying to enlighten people. Researchers have suggested that about ten to fifteen percent of people have auditory hallucinations and that, for many, this isn't a problem and they don't need intervention from mental health services. I, personally, have never had true auditory hallucinations, apart from very occasionally and non-specifically: some years ago I had an interesting evening when the unplugged radio busily played slightly badly tuned music for hours. So, it's pretty difficult to explain the goblin experience even now, and I still can't really get to the bottom of it twenty years on. No wonder I was permanently confused. Perhaps it was this permanent sense of confusion that engendered the unembroidered direct commands so loved by the goblins, as a sort of counterbalance to everything else about them, which was mostly inexplicable.

I would, truthfully, tell people, 'Yes, I know exactly what the goblins sound like, and, yes, they speak to me.' In fact, they actually sounded pretty much as I'd expect (funny that, I wonder what I'd have thought if they'd chosen a squeaky Birmingham voice?); essentially like creaky, wheezy, sinister, nasty, little old men. They were accentless too, which would have fitted in well with my belief systems, i.e. they were not tied to the northern town I was living in and they were authoritarian. But this was in my head; they were never heard externally by me. People would ask, 'How do you know what they sound like, if you can't really hear them?' And, 'If you don't hear them, then they're in your imagination, then?' What could I say? They were not in my head, not outside my head, not in my mind's eye or ear, not a product of my imagination … but a strange amalgam of all of these. It was almost another way of communication, unique to them and their magical powers. Sometimes, their audible words were posted into my head, ready-made, as though they were written on banners in red … sort of. Other times, not so much. It's all totally mystifying, even now. I knew exactly what they said. I just wasn't quite sure how they said it.

However, it was, and is, really difficult to explain, but there were some goblin manifestations that were definitely outside my head. They were present as a disturbance in the air, a cold breath, a weight against the ear. The goblin voice may or may not have been internal but the physicality of their speech was definitely external. Sometimes, they would sit upon my left shoulder, and I could feel their communication in my left ear but I couldn't actually hear it as an external voice. The voice was inside my head, but as far as I was concerned, it came from an external source. I don't know why they preferred the left, although, possibly coincidentally, I have slightly better hearing in that ear and the left is also traditionally known as the 'sinister' side.

It was the same with visual hallucinations, or rather non-hallucinations. I knew exactly what goblins looked like; there were the two basic, unvarying types of different sizes, but the smaller ones tended to be a bit bluer than the larger ones. The little ones were more imp-like, and comparatively rare after the early days. These were the little goblins who lived in cracks in the wall, and tended to manifest themselves as a meaningless bundle of nasty, but unintelligible, chatter.

I could sense both types of goblin outside me and had a powerful feeling of being constantly watched, whether they were 'visible' or not. When I saw goblins all around me, I think, or would like to think, that I suspected that they were some kind of inner generation and not a true hallucination. Visually, they weren't entirely solid; they were more slightly ethereal, perhaps ghost-like. Therefore they *should* have been a product of my mind's eye or imagination but, at the time, I was convinced that they weren't. My mind's eye or imagination, the most obvious culprits were, I believed, totally under my control, whereas those tricksy goblins were most certainly not under my control at all and appeared all over the place. Although the goblins were motionless when I looked at them, I firmly believed that they moved around freely when my back was turned, at all times of the day and night, and I also firmly believed that they enjoyed full and active lives without me.

So, where did that leave me? The two positions are fundamentally irreconcilable. If goblins were phantoms internally generated by me, they could hardly enjoy active, external lives totally without me. I certainly didn't believe that I was creating goblins internally, and then somehow (rather nastily) wishing them on the world at large. That wouldn't have made any sense to me at all, as goblin folklore predates my own goblin obsession by hundreds of years. There really wasn't much joy when I tried to explain the situation to other people.

The only indisputably real hallucinations I had were hypnagogic, which are harmless and common. Somewhere, in the borderlands between sleep and wakefulness, I would feel the bed shake, and I would be prodded by sharp goblin fingers. This was the only time when goblins had any corporeality and I found it terrifying.

The physical inner workings of the goblin body were, to me, a total mystery. They were humanoid and appeared very old, and probably enjoyed some form of eternal life, as befitted the godlike status I afforded them. I also, usually, envisaged them with cold, reptilian blood and dank, leathery skin. However, I never proved, or disproved, this last theory, as I always attempted to keep goblins as well away from me as possible, and certainly never attempted to touch them. Not only was I too scared, but it would have also felt somewhat impolite.

However, back with the indisputably real, I did get an unpleasant wallop of reality which I couldn't dismiss. I brought this on myself, and it was like a bomb in my quiet little world where I had, I now suspect, been somewhat sheltered by Dr R. In 2000 medical information was not easily accessible like it is today. I certainly didn't have access to encouraging websites that discussed illnesses, medication, prognosis, rights and all the rest. 'Take this test and see if you'd better take yourself off to the doctor as soon as possible,' might pop up in the medical pages of a women's magazine, but I didn't read those anymore. I'd actually only ever read free copies in launderettes, and, 'I did my facelift with a staple gun' (fact, apparently) was a bit gothic even for me. It surely indicated some form of mental illness, but it wasn't one I could relate to.

So, finding out information felt rather like a trip to the woods to find blackberries. I'd go off full of purpose, search about a bit, hope the ones I discovered weren't sour (i.e. wrong) and very possibly draw a total blank. In other words, once I'd exhausted the limited information provided by medical professionals, information gathering was a haphazard and hazardous task.

I was no further forward than the 'psychosis' definition on the blood test form and there must have been some sort of a patient information leaflet with the medication but, overall, there wasn't a lot to go on. For all my brave thoughts, I was deeply conflicted. I wanted to know what was going on, and I didn't want to know what was going on. Eventually, one afternoon, when I was officially at work, I accessed my small well of courage and decided to visit the local reference library - an illicit excursion, as private psychosis investigation was hardly in my job description. If anybody had asked, or even noticed, I would have said I was doing some research, which was truthful; it just wasn't work related research. After some rather random wandering about (I was too embarrassed to ask for the insanity shelf), I ended up with the 'P' volume of the *Encyclopaedia Britannica*. P is for psychosis. Obviously.

I opened it up surreptitiously - I did not want to be seen reading about psychosis - and found a quiet corner of the library with a view of the busy street beyond. I have no idea how the *Encyclopaedia Britannica* discusses psychosis today, but the volume I found in 2000 was a profoundly alarming and depressing read. I gathered that I seemed to have started along a one-way path of devastating mental and social deterioration. The ultimate destination was not clearly elucidated, but my competent imagination filled in the gaps. My condition appeared to be a sort of terminal illness of the mind and soul, and I'd eventually be left with a functioning body and not much else. I felt sick and my heart was pounding. I'd have given anything to be one of those ordinary shoppers outside, to be in their present world and not in the horrible one that seemed to have ambushed me.

After a few minutes, I persevered grimly. I now came across something I'd never heard of or read about before: **delusions of control**. These, so-called, 'delusions of control' were horribly familiar. 'I've got goblins telling me what to do.' I'd been telling everyone. 'And quite often I do it.' Oh dear. Delusions of control were apparently typically found in schizophrenia. This was, genuinely, the first time I'd considered the schizophrenia diagnosis. Like everyone else, I knew all about schizophrenia. Basically you were a *schizo*. It meant you had ridiculous hallucinations and went round waving an axe, or some such, in a deranged and blood thirsty manner. WTF! I can't put it more strongly even now. Anyway, I didn't even own an axe. I'd got the wrong kind of garden; it was minuscule. I mentally slid over the business of hallucinations, hmm, yes, well goblins ... possibly. But my goblins, though unpleasant, hadn't told me to hurt anyone else.

At the next appointment, I asked Dr R if I'd got schizophrenia. She said she didn't think so; it was probably something more transitory, as I'd responded well to treatment. I felt ashamed and embarrassed that I'd asked, as though I was suffering from a form of over-dramatic, mental hypochondria. So, I never asked her again. When she moved on, more than six months later, I still didn't know I had schizophrenia, but everybody else did.

I'm not sure why this diagnosis was kept from me. I'm guessing it was kindly meant as a form of protection, but it left me very confused. OK, I wasn't doing at all well in establishing a constructive, therapeutic relationship with Dr R, and this was largely down to me, but tip-toeing around my diagnosis really wasn't very helpful. As far as I was concerned, my medical problems remained nameless and vague and by implication what? Minor? Insubstantial? Made up? Hysterical? This wasn't how I was being treated, so I was receiving very mixed messages indeed.

For over a year, all the clinic letters about me - which, of course, I didn't see at the time - carried the warning that my paranoid schizophrenia diagnosis had not been discussed with me, so, 'nobody mention it, please'. Absolutely nobody did, which is pretty impressive. When I finally returned to the schizophrenia question again, asking a different psychiatrist this time, he told me, 'yes, you do have schizophrenia.' I still cried after I left his consulting room, as it confirmed so much, although it wasn't, by now, a great surprise. But why was it down to me to initiate that conversation? I was, after all, a grown up and, outside my run-ins with the claustrophobic and coercive medical world, I was living independently. If I hadn't plucked up the courage to ask again, when was anyone planning to tell me? Or did everyone hope it was someone else's unhappy job?

It was unintentionally counterproductive, as my unnamed and, to me, unidentified problems were so much more difficult for me to mentally ring-fence and inspect. Knowing what was wrong might ... possibly ... have helped with the goblins. I saw them as my unique problem, probably correct in one narrow way, and not, more broadly, as part of an illness. Hence, I tended to evaluate help using dodgy criteria. I'd ask, 'How can you help fix goblins? Nobody, but me, seems to know anything about goblins,' when I should have been asking: 'How can you help fix my illness?' Mental health services know all about schizophrenia, it's a common enough problem: about one percent of us will suffer from it at some point during our lifetime. But, perhaps, it would have made no difference; it was a very long time indeed until I really understood that goblins were only symptoms, and not the illness itself.

Meanwhile, I limped on at work. Looking back, my manager was remarkably kind and tolerant. At the time, I was very worried that the goblins were coming into the building via the basement drainage system. I legitimately worked in this basement (as well as having a desk in the main office) as it was the home of the museum's main art store. Some years ago, there had been some kind of flooding so, logically, I thought, there must be a secret network of drains underneath the town and they probably linked up together. It would be easy for a goblin to enter the drains at my home and surreptitiously make their way to the museum. At work, I selected the most obvious basement drain and wrote: 'Beware, goblins' in very small letters, on the plastic flooring. This, I hoped, would have some kind of talismanic significance, perhaps protective. It certainly made me feel less irresponsible. I was warning people, wasn't I?

I also strongly considered writing a similar message on the staff information whiteboard but, luckily, a powerful instinct for self-preservation meant I didn't go through with this. However, every working day started with a battle. 'Is this the day,' I'd ask myself, 'that I am brave and strong, and warn my colleagues about the dangers of goblindom?' Or, alternatively, 'Is this the day I enlighten my colleagues about the magnificent, messianic goblins?' Very fairy tale language. The goblins were extremely enthusiastic about the 'magnificent, messianic' idea. They also encouraged me to take out advertisements in newspapers and share the word, so to speak, in the town's main square. Fortunately, I was too timid.

Unfortunately I'd started amending, while still taking, the antipsychotic dose, to fit in with my lifestyle and my perceptions of who I was. As I hadn't got that alarming condition, schizophrenia, but something vaguely on the spectrum but milder, I was increasingly intolerant of the inconveniences of my illness. I was learning the well-recorded downside of antipsychotics, which work by damping down brain activity and so left me apathetic and exhausted. Who was this new person? There were parts of her I didn't recognise at all. I really didn't think very highly of her. It was all very frustrating.

For a while, I had been fairly resigned to the situation. After all, I'd only be taking the medication for a few weeks, wouldn't I? My life would then return to normal, wouldn't it? When I mentioned this optimistic assumption to Sean, I learned, to my horror, that antipsychotics weren't usually prescribed like this. I would be taking them for, at the very least, six months to a year, and that was if I was one of the lucky ones. 'Hang on a sec ...' I thought, 'I'm going to have to live in this bleak, flat, exhausted world for how long? I've got things to do. How am I going to manage big projects at work?' And, more pertinently, 'How am I going to have a life at all?'

Sadly, this wasn't a question I should have been asking at all but hindsight is, famously, a fine thing. What if? What if? The 'what if?' game. What if I had taken the medication as prescribed properly, and not just at the beginning? What if I'd accepted more of what I was told and learned from all those people who tried to help? Why did I insist on continuing to fight them when I had nothing much left to lose? Why was I such a bad patient, when I was the one who kept getting hurt? Would I have had one discrete episode, and then my life would have returned to relative normality? I'd be a bit battered, but considerably wiser, and definitely more able to manage my mental health. That's something I'll never know, and it hurts to write about it.

It's clear from my notes, that, as spring went on, things started to slide dramatically, and this was not just because I was more honest in the consultations. My intellectual skills were deteriorating, especially my ability to express myself verbally. I was finding it increasingly difficult to explain my predicament, particularly when talking directly about goblins. In the letter below, it is described as having 'no words.' So, a couple of times, I wrote things down. This had always been my preferred method of communication in any case.

This is a transcription of a letter I wrote to Sean, dated 17th May 2000. It is in my medical notes, which is why I have access to it now. It was written off the cuff, with minimal alterations. My handwriting, which I barely recognise, is terrible, so I don't know if it was fully read. In the transcription I've made a couple of deletions where there are personal names, which appear as ...'They' refers to goblins, and I've also specifically not named the town.

Dear Sean

I hope this reaches you before you go on leave. It is being written entirely illegally at work, but I am a bit stuck (can't think of a more appropriate word) and didn't want to talk to you directly (no words). I am not taking the sulpiride and have no plans to do so before the next appointment with Dr R. It is living death taking it, they don't like it, and anyway if I don't take it, it is much easier to keep on top of what they are up to. I don't know how to tell people at work but they are everywhere. But you can't go talking about them because saying you believe in goblins is in most people's eyes, tantamount to saying you talk to fridges (which I don't.) But that's not to say that they aren't <u>*very dangerous*</u>*, and there are a lot of them in the ... store where ... goes. And I ought to tell him as they might get at him, and he might not know. And I can't tell my line manager because she wouldn't recognise one if it leapt up and bit her. They live in pot plants, + under desks, + in other corners. They used to just live in my head in Autumn, but now this year I've realised quite how many of them there are, all over .... (outside? ...) and quite how much power they have. But I haven't the courage to warn people, which is very weak willed on my part. What damage this can cause, I don't know. I am finding living with the responsibility very difficult. It gets in the way of work because*

it is so much more important than work if only people realised, but they don't + I don't think I've got the ability to make them understand, + the risks they are taking.
Anyway, I hope you are well, and sorry to land you with such an illegible scrawl, but I am rather overwhelmed ...

A quick explanatory note in my defence. The pot plant bit, which sounds suspiciously humorous, was actually sensible within my world view. Goblins had an affinity for natural places in most fairyland accounts. Therefore, if they were infiltrating the office where I worked, any form of greenery would be as close as they could get to their natural habitat. Hence also their liking for nice, wet drains.

This letter provides an alternative reasoning for the medication rejection. Goblins don't like medication. They don't like it one little bit. It interrupts their lines of communication, and that's a bad thing. Isn't it? Then there's me. I don't like it either; it affects my performance at work, quite apart from the rest of my life. So, the goblins and I were in agreement here, the actual reasoning about medication non-compliance might be different but the end result was the same.

Overall, I am curious about my concern for the well-being of others here. It's not something I remember, except in the vaguest of ways, so it can't have lasted long. I wonder whether this apparent concern was actually expressing the escalating level of threat and danger that I felt endangered me, rather than any actual anxieties for anyone else. Certainly, the goblins were on a trajectory of nastiness. First, I was told to do things. Then I was threatened if I didn't comply. Now other people were being threatened too though they were, unsurprisingly, totally unaware of the danger they were in.

This cry for help letter got a speedy response. I was apparently offered admission to hospital, which I rejected, and my medication was changed to olanzapine. At the time, I was also apparently very concerned that the goblins were plotting something nasty, but unspecified, possibly on quite a wide scale.

I wish I could say that things stabilised. But they didn't and, to my distress, I too was emerging as a threat. The goblins and I were creating an unholy partnership. I guess it was inevitable really. How many of my subsequent delusions and hallucinations were conditioned because I'd chosen goblins? I expected goblins to be malevolent because that's their role in fairyland. Therefore, they were malevolent.

I can't remember anything at all about what was written below, but it's worth noting that I really liked the friend and, largely because we had written some museum related, non-fiction together, we had a trusting relationship. 12th June 2000. Written by Sean:

> *On Sunday went to visit her friend ... Prior to this Jane had contacted her and explained that she had a psychotic illness, her friend was accepting of this and invited her down. This was at the suggestion of Dr R as Jane has told no-one and does not want to tell her family ... Apparently the visit went well ... On the way home the 'Gnomes' told Jane that she had to destroy the friend and the best way was to kill her friends yet unborn baby. Jane was very alarmed re their statement. When Jane was discussing these with me I got the impression she was intimating to me to tell her not to act on these thoughts ... this I did and she felt immediately better and told me that is what she wanted me to do ...*

It was a good response from Sean here, and it reminds me why I valued him. It was an early warning sign of trouble and at this stage fairly fleeting. I could still be reassured that these violent thoughts were abnormal and unreasonable, more suggestions than commands. But the balance of power was continuing to shift. Who was increasingly in charge now? It sounds suspiciously as though it might have been the goblins (emphatically not gnomes, Sean).

So off I went, medicated again, and relatively sane for the next couple of weeks. Looking at my notes, I seem to have been attending the previously spurned day hospital but only first thing in the morning to take medication. But then I stopped the medication again ... and the goblins were now threatening to kill me if I took any medication at all. My ability to function plummeted and I was, of course, unable to go to work. When Sean visited, he said he was concerned, but was, as ever, polite, helpful and encouraging - whatever he might have been actually thinking inside.

Conversations went on behind my back about enforced hospital admission, if I continued to refuse medication, under the 1983 Mental Health Act. I apparently had, 'some lucid states', which, I should imagine, were when I was not talking repetitively about evil, homicidal, all-controlling goblins. It was, presumably, during one of these lucid states that Sean informed me of the sectioning process, which I'd heard of but didn't understand, believing that you were only sectioned if you were suicidal. But I wasn't suicidal at all. Yes, the goblins were very keen on having me dead, but I wasn't so sure that I agreed with them. Sean warned me that, if at all possible, I should avoid being sectioned as it would be legally on my record forever. It was the only bit of advice I heeded.

Sean was away for the rest of a week, so I was visited by a couple of other members of the team. They were perfectly pleasant and well-motivated, but, according to my medical notes, I referred to them as, 'the community psychiatric police', so I don't think I welcomed their visits. Things were getting increasingly serious for me and I was being monitored daily, whether I liked it or not. On Friday, one of these nurses turned up again on my doorstep. I, presumably somewhat warily, let her in (I don't remember this bit at all) but there is suddenly a crystal clear, jagged sliver of memory, cutting across my brain.

'Take your medication, take it now!' she shouted, effectively trapping me against the stairs.

I was shocked and stunned. What had just happened? Why was I being shouted at by a virtual stranger in my own home? I wasn't angry, just frozen and bewildered. Nobody from mental health services had startled me with this approach before.

They'd informed me of some uncomfortable facts, but had never spoken to me so forcibly. I was used to the carefully expressed language of therapy, not such direct and alarming honesty. Now, the normal adult conventions of civilised confrontation seemed to have totally evaporated. It didn't occur to me that it was a last ditch attempt to keep me out of hospital, so it was for my own benefit.

Did it work? No, I still refused to take the medication, in spite of everything I'd been told by everybody - again and again and again. My brain had totally seized up. I couldn't see any further ahead than not taking medication, nothing at all. How did I think I was going to manage going forward? Was it all up to the goblins? In the 'real' world, I couldn't go to work, or sleep and had barely eaten. Was this really a viable lifestyle?

The nurse gave me an unequivocal ultimatum. If I didn't take medication I would have to be taken to the hospital. Now. If I didn't go willingly, I would be sectioned. No ifs, no buts. I had a stark choice. As taking the medication was an impossibility for me, I had to accept hospital admission. Stupefied me could give no thought whatsoever, to what this might entail. I hadn't actually made a decision as such; I'd just refused the sensible option and now had to live with the consequences.

It was all deeply confusing. Even more of my everyday normality appeared to have suddenly vanished. What was happening to my life? Had I entered a parallel universe? (Leaving aside the goblin parallel universe which was far less parallel and more integrated with me than I would have liked). What I thought about hospital admission ... NO!! ... was clearly irrelevant, even though it was me who was going to have to go there. How had thirty one year old me, most definitely grown up and living a grown up life, suddenly and unwillingly regressed to childhood? Or had taken, without my knowledge, to some kind of punishable criminal lifestyle? Either way, I was shocked by this sudden, entirely legal, deprivation of my liberty. Yes, I knew it could happen in principle, I'd been amply warned about it, but those warnings were, only now, beginning to sink in.

I vaguely gathered together some possessions as requested, but I didn't end up taking much more than a toothbrush. It was all too much mental effort to sort out what I should be packing, and I didn't plan to stay a minute longer at the hospital than I had to. I was a voluntary patient, wasn't I? I knew what 'voluntary' meant. It meant you were doing something of your own free will. I was wearing some awful old clothes I wore around the house for DIY and dirty jobs, but it didn't occur to me to change them. Normally, I wouldn't have let a psychiatric nurse see me in these clothes, let alone go out in public, but I'd forgotten that I was wearing them.

It was a lovely Friday evening. The streets of the town were full of people celebrating the end of the working week and generally enjoying the sunshine. But I wasn't. I was being taken against my will to somewhere I really didn't want to go. My weekend was not looking promising at all. When we arrived at the psychiatric unit we turned left, and went up some stairs to the female ward. It was the first time I'd seen this part of the building. The most positive interpretation I could make of the matter, was that the hospital staff were unlikely to try to kill me - whereas the murderous goblins had entirely different ideas.

CHAPTER 7 INVOLUNTARY VOLUNTARY

At the hospital, I sat on the bed and cried a little. It was the first time I'd cried for months and it was a weird feeling. I wasn't crying solely because I was at the hospital; my few tears were for the whole ghastly mess. In spite of all the warnings, I hadn't really understood that the psychiatric ward actually existed. But it did and here I was, indisputably.

What had just happened? In my experience of mental illness people were generally depressed and/or stressed, took some pills, had some time off work, then life for them resumed roughly as normal. Why hadn't my mental illness, if I had one, been treated the same way? It certainly didn't mean being metaphorically picked up by the hair, whirled around a few times and ending up dumped in a hospital, just because I wouldn't take a few pills. Surely, the matter of pill taking was my decision, wasn't it? It was my life after all. I was a grown up, wasn't I? It was all deeply unfair and confusing. Why had I been singled out for this unpleasant, special treatment? What had I said, or done, that was so wrong?

A round of form filling ensued and probably some kind of orientation but, as I was only partly with it, not a great deal went in. As a result, I was about to spend quite a lot of time on the ward learning the routine by watching other people, basically so that I didn't get told off. It was, I discovered, very easy to get told off as a patient on a psychiatric ward. This was hardly surprising, as we were patients precisely because we'd failed to live up to our status as grown ups. We were in a state of childish dependency.

In due course, it was time to see the senior on-call house officer. These are extracts from his notes, 23rd June 2000:

She presented very withdrawn and aloof. Initially she wouldn't say more than 'I want to go home' and remained silent for about 25 minutes. She refused a stat dose of olanzapine 10mg. On further prompt she admitted to hearing voices by 'goblins' telling her 'You will die if you take the medication'. She also added that these goblins are everywhere, they know what she thinks and are telling her she is evil and should harm her friend's baby after birth. She admitted to being terrified of the 'goblins' and their 'powers'. She expressed feelings of hopelessness and helplessness stating 'I can't see any future' ...

MSE revealed a 31 yrs old lady dressed in dirty clothes (evidence of neglect) who appeared rather frightened and made very poor eye contact. Her speech was diminished in volume and poor in content - she used mostly monosyllabic answers. Her mood was objectively and subjectively low and anxious with flattened affect. There was evidence of delusions of control, persecutory delusions and passivity phenomena ('the goblins control my actions'). It is worth mentioning that these delusional beliefs were not unshakeable. She admitted hearing or feeling in an extrasensorial way 'the goblins' and described experience resembling depersonalisation. She denied to answer questions regarding self harm thoughts ... Her cognitive functions were within normal limits on gross testing. She partly believed that these experiences can be attributed to a mental illness ...

I spent twenty five minutes in a state of hostile, almost complete silence? I've edited this bit from my memory totally, so reading this account was an unpleasant surprise. Eventually, I accepted the medication, believing this would mean I would be discharged. Taking the medication was the only bit of the interview I remembered. It stayed with me, as it was such a humiliating memory. The doctor went through all the usual sensible reasons as to why it might be a good idea. Well, I'd heard these endlessly from various people, so we didn't get very far.

Eventually, as a last resort, he decided to join me in fantasy land. Interestingly enough, he didn't record this in the notes.

This may be because mental health workers generally try to avoid getting too caught up in a patient's delusional world. They really don't want to be inadvertently validating it. Consequently, they are rather fond of the statement: 'I believe that you believe (insert delusion of choice).' Ouch. This was a statement I grew to hate over the years. I understand why mental health types use it, but it is a bit patronising when you're on the receiving end. Then again, how would I manage a determinedly delusional patient? I suspect that whatever you try, you can't win, which must be deeply discouraging.

This particular doctor, no doubt desperately, decided to jettison the normal rules, hence the silence in my notes. I forget the exact details, so the following is a very rough reconstruction. Apparently, there was some kind of battle going on in my brain between the forces of good and evil, and this was very important. It could affect the world. The goblins didn't like medication, as they were evil, but they definitely couldn't kill me. However, I wasn't evil, and the medication would help the good part of my brain battle on.

Nobody had tried this particular argument before and it captured my attention. Was taking the medication part of a wider social good? It was not just me it would be helping? Was I caught in a battle between good and evil? 'Quite possibly,' I thought. So, I swallowed the pill (as well as the argument), and the poor, no doubt exhausted doctor sighed and relaxed. I noticed this relaxation but at the time I didn't understand it; I hadn't even noticed that he was tense in the first place. I'd given absolutely no thought whatsoever to the intellectual and emotional pressure he'd been under even though we'd been locked in combat for a very long time.

'Can I go home now?' I asked optimistically.

His answer was, 'No.'

Over the next few days, in spite of goblin threats, I showed no signs of dying. The goblins, of course, had an answer to this. 'We didn't mean literal physical death,' (goblin eye roll if they were capable of such things), 'we meant the death of the soul, the death of your brain. You belong to us.'

'They could well be right about that,' I thought despairingly.

I yearned for my home, where it was quiet and private and my bedroom was dark and cool. Where I wasn't trying to live and sleep in a boiling hot, restless, noisy public place. At home, nobody cared about what I did or didn't do and I wasn't anxiously trying to conform to a set of ward behavioural rules that I hadn't quite mastered. I could also change my clothes - I was still wearing the unfortunate ones I was admitted in - and it was even more important as my period started. In the upset of the last few days, I had forgotten it was due. I was too shy to ask for sanitary protection and my clothes were, by now, all bloodied anyway. At least the dreadful trousers were black, so no one noticed.

My whereabouts were constantly checked and I had no idea why. It's not nice being inspected at the best of times, and I found it alarming and annoying. No one told me that I was considered an absconsion risk. I discovered this much later, from my medical notes, and also that the staff tried to minimise the checks on me because I was 'frightened'. They were right; I was frightened and I can see from the notes that on that first night, I 'slept' (it was very fragmentary) in my clothes, too scared to undress.

I had no idea what the plan was for me over the next few days and, as it was the weekend, there was no opportunity to find out. Nobody seemed to know anything much or, if they did, they weren't sharing it with me. I didn't understand that my medical plan would be worked out by my usual psychiatrist - Dr R - after the weekend, so I was totally lost and bewildered.

After a while, I took matters into my own hands and announced: 'Thanks very much and all that, but as I'm a voluntary patient, I'm off. Bye!' This caused a flap and I learned that I needed medical approval to leave. This was puzzling and disquieting but, as I believed that I was admitted because of medication non-compliance and I was now obediently taking the medication (for all of twenty four hours), I couldn't see any reasons to detain me. I recall being reasonably calm and sensible during this exchange. However, the nursing notes described me as being 'distressed and irritable', so I think I must have ironed out my recollections somewhat.

A very long time later (so it felt), I was interviewed by another junior doctor, and I put forward my case. If I couldn't be discharged, could I, at least, have a few hours home leave please? After a telephone call to the on-call consultant, I was recalled to the consulting room. There was no home leave allowed and, if I tried to go, I would be sectioned. You what? So basically, it was the same as the admission process; 'voluntary', yet again, meant no such thing. I was an involuntary voluntary patient. Or vice versa. I was very disappointed, and also furious, as I had been picturing myself in my peaceful home. It had never seemed so attractive. Why couldn't I, at the very least, have got some clean clothes? I'd have come back, wouldn't I? (Hmm ... would I?) Why was I incarcerated in this prison-like place, anyway? I hadn't committed a crime, had I? All I did was refuse to take some small white pills.

I had learned a valuable lesson. You don't mess with mental health services because they have powers, genuine legal powers. Just like the police. I was increasingly regarding them as interchangeable. I never refused medication again, at least not so adamantly. There were many times when I was medication non-compliant but, when my back was against the wall and I was threatened with the dreaded hospital, I would capitulate. My worldview was increasingly bleak. I seemed to be at the bottom of an authoritarian vertical hierarchy: goblins on top, mental health services underneath, and what was left of me, most definitely right at the bottom, somehow clinging on and with no hope of moving upwards.

Some days later, I saw Dr R. It took a while, as it transpired she worked part time. At least she wasn't on holiday. If she had been, would I have had to wait until she returned? I was determined to escape this horrible place, so I gave the kind of bravura performance I normally reserved for job interviews. I was intent on convincing her that I was perfectly all right to go home. Also, that I had been chastened by my hospital experience - this much was true, and I would in future be a model patient, take the medication and re-join normal life as soon as possible. Simple.

I'm not quite sure I entirely believed this upbeat script, and it was pretty obvious Dr R was somewhat dubious, although she did describe me as more 'biddable' in my notes (not a usual description of an adult. What was I? A mistrustful Shetland pony?) I was, unfortunately, like the reformed prisoner on the brink of release, full of hopeful high ideals and determined not to slip back into the bad old ways. Yet I was going back to the same environment that helped cause my crime, if you could call it that, in the first place. I didn't secure my immediate discharge and I was not given a concrete release date. My bravura performance had failed. Although I was given increasing concessions, and spent more and more time at home, it was two weeks until I was properly discharged. I vowed never to come back.

Sadly, it's pretty clear from my notes that this new responsible, 'biddable' me, didn't last long and I was soon back to my medication-avoiding old ways, with little real understanding of the extent to which I was damaging my health and, rather more holistically, my life. I'm not sure to what extent I cared anyway. By now, I regarded myself as a thoroughly evil person and was mystified as to why people treated me kindly, as though I were some form of normal human being. So, if the people around me weren't trying to hurt me, I'd better compensate and hurt myself. As well as being definitely evil, I still regarded myself as deeply feeble and this was my secondary crime. I was intensely frustrated at my inability to get on top of the situation.

I eagerly swallowed accounts of 'how to live without medication', and how it was just a question of clean living and positive mental attitude. I gazed wistfully and enviously at people who'd mastered their serious psychiatric issues, so much more serious than mine. They had abandoned coercive medication and were now living fulfilled, spiritually harmonious and productive lives. Or thereabouts. My intellectual vanity assured me that, as an intelligent person, it should be something I could achieve too. What was the problem?

It was an eternally elusive ambition. I enjoyed the physical and emotional rush I experienced when I abandoned medication, and a feeling that I was in touching distance of my old self. This was also when I experienced blinding revelations about the goblin world, how it was structured and, potentially, how it could be managed. My blinding revelations were usually, well, wrong ... but I saw them as important and essential moments of spiritual enlightenment. Without these moments, that is when I was medicated, I worried incessantly about missing the various sinister happenings in the goblin world. This wilful blindness could be very dangerous, or so I believed.

I also refused to accept that antipsychotic medication, while not addictive, does change the way the brain works, therefore I would not automatically return to my pre-medication (just about) functioning state. So invariably, when unmedicated, I soon wore myself out. I was totally unable to sleep, my brain would be wound up so tightly it froze, and I would be completely in thrall to the goblins, and, once they were aware, increasingly harried by an exasperated mental health services. Any new insights into the goblin world would always turn out to be, at best, pointless and, at worst, dangerous, but I seemed to be particularly obtuse when it came to recognising this inevitably unhappy scenario or at modifying my behaviour to avoid it.

All this time, I'd been going to work, resolutely acting normally, or so I hoped, but not achieving much. I'd told my manager, on several occasions, about the goblins in the Art Store, probably because I couldn't stand the secrecy anymore and also for reassurance. It was a lonely world with goblins, as nobody ever agreed with me. 'Please just give me the tiniest window of comfort,' I thought of everyone. 'Just the tiniest bit of belief.' But, of course, there was never any belief on offer. Why would there be? My manager would look uncomfortable and tell me that, 'there really aren't goblins in the basement.' End of conversation on that point. Well, that's how I remember it. My manager told me, subsequently, that she didn't deny the reality of the goblins and she may be right, although her embarrassed and anxious silence was pretty telling. Poor woman; she hadn't signed up to be a mental health professional. I, however, felt extremely misunderstood at the time. Goblins in the Art Store was a major problem for the museum, and certainly not something to be ignored and denied. What had happened to free speech? Why was I being suppressed? Luckily, there was a tiny part of me that considered my pronouncements to be odd and possibly, perhaps, not quite right. Thank goodness for that small inner moderating critic; it tended to protect me from the kind of announcements or deeds that would otherwise have landed me in serious trouble. I was, by this time, feeling totally overwhelmed and isolated at work and apparently, according to my medical notes, I asked to resign again. However, this was seen as a welfare issue, and I was told to take sick leave for a couple of weeks instead.

The goblins, destructive as ever when it came to my well-being, were extremely keen for me to leave work and sell the house. However, they hadn't really provided an alternative plan, other than for me to go to the top of a local, multi-storey car park and jump off. They assured me that I could fly. I, usually, correctly regarded the flying part as another goblin trick to get me to kill myself. After all, if I really believed I could fly, I'd have dashed over to the car park to give it a go - what an exhilarating skill to have! Could goblins themselves fly? I don't think I asked them, but it was possible, as they enjoyed all sorts of special powers. However, even with goblin help, I knew my supernatural powers were non-existent. (Apart, of course, from the tricky issue of goblins, which I didn't perceive as supernatural at all, whatever a more broad-minded observer might think.)

After two weeks, I returned to work, but it didn't go well. There is a total blank in my memory as to what went on; in fact I'd entirely erased the whole unhappy incident, so it was a surprise when I found it in my notes. What happened? What did I say? Or do? Whatever it was, my manager at work must have had the number of the community mental health team; I must have been asked for it as I can't see how they would have it otherwise. This next bit is from my medical notes:

31st July 2000. Out of hours service referral/action form. Sean was presumably away, but I recognise the handwriting. It was completed by the lucky team member who'd previously taken me to hospital.

... received a call from ... saying that they were extremely concerned about Jane's behaviour at work ... Visited this evening. Somewhat hostile towards our visit but allowed us in. Jane was shocked and angry ...

I'm not surprised I was shocked and angry. I don't think work had told me that they'd called the mental health team, so all of this was a deeply unpleasant surprise. By thinking and thinking and thinking, I can dredge up a few vague recollections, and I believe that I'd simply gone home as normal at the end of the working day. There was absolutely no way I was allowed to return to work the following day, especially as a sick note had already been arranged for me. It was a fait accompli.

At the time, I thought it a very underhand way for work to behave. How would they like it? I didn't give any consideration as to the relatively gentle way it was handled. I wasn't exactly marched off the premises, but I really didn't think I'd actually done anything, or said anything too dreadful, had I? It was deeply disturbing because I'd clearly progressed, or perhaps regressed, from, 'troubled but basically not too bad with leeway,' to, 'so out of touch with reality that is not safe to have around the place ...' It was not something that had ever happened to me before, in any shape or form. My previously orderly life was progressively more and more baffling and disorderly.

The unfortunate mental health team members also visited on 3rd of August, apparently. However, according to their notes, I wouldn't let them in at all. I imagine we had some sort of low level standoff on the doorstep. I'm not sure why; perhaps I was blaming them for the work debacle, or maybe I just didn't want to talk. Unfortunately, 'don't shoot the messenger' as a concept doesn't seem to have crossed my mind. My unwanted visitors would probably have been quite helpful.

The enforced sick leave, to be perfectly honest, was a relief. My concentration remained appalling. I spent the summer drifting round the house and the town, in an irresolute manner. I went to the day hospital on weekdays, but only to take medication there, so I could outmanoeuvre the goblins. Nobody made me stay any longer. (Weekend medication taking was more patchy.) I told mental health services that I didn't need more than the brief morning visits to the day hospital because I was getting on with the decorating at home. This was a fib so they'd leave me alone. However regularly I set myself up in the back bedroom, full of somewhat manufactured determination, I soon lost focus and gave up. The house remained mostly stripped back. It wasn't very homely.

I felt deeply unhappy, dislocated, and hopeless, and was apparently still telling people the various violent ways the goblins had in mind for my suicide. Dr R, the psychiatrist, considered this to be a psychotic issue, not a depressive illness, so I wasn't offered antidepressants. I have no recorded opinions on this subject, and, as I was relatively medication naive, it never occurred to me that antidepressants might be a good idea.

Rather more worrying for everyone, was that I was still, sporadically, reporting the goblins' enthusiasm for baby killing. My friend's baby had now been born, and I believed I should take the baby's pram and push it under a bus. Dr R told me that I must not visit the friend, and that I also needed to tell her what was going on. I was sad about this, and nervous about destroying our friendship, especially as I didn't have many friends nearby in any case. This was my reaction, as dispassionately recorded in my notes. It's a pretty damning and uncomfortable read. I was obviously prioritising my needs for social companionship, and desire to save face, over the vital needs of a tiny, helpless child and his family.

That said, there was some logic behind my somewhat warped views and this was my own internal risk assessment. Firstly, I was well enough to understand potential consequences. I knew it was wrong to take a life and I understood how devastating it would be for everyone, were I to do so. Well, that's what I like to think, although I suspect that my grasp of these consequences was somewhat compromised. I was never able to think through, or even imagine, the immediate aftermath of a baby killing episode. Just imagine … I've killed a baby and am now standing over it, with its mother, both disbelieving and unbelievably distressed, nearby. How would I feel? What would I do? There'd be no waking up and finding it was all an awful dream. Yet again, the goblins were obscurely silent on this scenario.

I was on sounder ground when it came to the second consequence. I knew I'd end up somewhere like Broadmoor for a very long time indeed, whatever the goblins might have me believe. Threats of Broadmoor appear frequently in my notes, as it was obvious that while I might be somewhat careless of other people's rights, I was perfectly aware of my own. After my recent hospital experience, I was not in the least reconciled to the joys of an institutional lifestyle.

Thirdly, and thankfully, when I was actually with babies, especially if they were awake, my normal, maternal instincts kicked in. I was barely aware of this particular mechanism at the time; as far as I was concerned the baby was actively 'protecting' itself, rather as if it were aware that an agent of the evil goblins was hoping to kill it. I would kiss the top of its head, talk nonsense to it, dance it up and down - all the normal stuff. As a big sister, I already knew how to treat a baby, but it was more than a, 'I guess I'd better go through the normal repertoire ...' It was inbuilt.

Sadly, I wasn't fully aware of this natural response and how it worked. Hence, I frequently worried that it was in some way superficial and could be easily overridden by a combination of the goblins and my natural evil. After all, I was clearly an unnatural woman. This new discovery about myself was repulsive and condemnatory. I could understand that a persistently crying baby, while not deserving of harm, might inspire some unhappy thoughts in its carer, but my friend's baby had done nothing to me whatsoever. I couldn't claim he had been screaming for hours; we hadn't even met.

It was all very murky, and matters became even darker. These homicidal thoughts were only goblin punishments and warnings directed at me, weren't they? Me ... the unwilling centre of everything. I, *myself,* didn't want to harm the baby at all. I was quite fond of babies. Why was I being held responsible for vile goblin plots? It wasn't fair. The worst you could say about me is that I had been selected by goblins for my evil potential ... which was admittedly problematic, as this evil potential seemed to be developing nicely... Goblins were very tricky customers: they lied, they manipulated, they were past masters at changing the goal posts, they threatened and they punished. But did they really kill? Did they really want me to kill? Or was it some diabolical kind of game? People kept telling me that goblins weren't real. How could they make me kill someone? Why were people worried that I could kill this child, when they were so keen to make me disavow the goblins? If people believed goblins didn't exist, how could they believe that these non-existent beings were telling me what to do? But goblins *are* real, aren't they?

These thoughts went round and round in my head. The above paragraph is meant to read as though it's in a washing machine on a spin cycle; that's what it felt like. I find it odd, reading about command hallucinations in fiction and in the news, that they are often presented as almost psychopathically, emotionally empty. My commands might have been unembellished, and thus straight to the point, but a huge amount of emotion, energy and confusion was bound up in them. Nothing was at all straightforward. I was usually bewildered and couldn't see a way through at all. This, I'm guessing, is the 'thought disorder' described in my medical notes. When it came to babies I vacillated between:

> 'I am an evil baby killer.'
>
> 'I am a friend, sort of, of the goblins, probably selected for my magnificent evil baby killing potential ...'
>
> 'I am an unfortunate and innocent person, who has been singled out for the kind of goblin attention I could really do without.'
>
> 'I am ill.'

This last option was very popular with medical professionals, but was usually, but not always, dismissed by me. It wasn't for want of trying by the aforementioned medical types.

The word 'disingenuous' did not occur to me at all, though some years later I met a psychologist who was very keen on it indeed. I really don't seem to have had any awareness that if nasty goblins weren't thinking up all these plans, somebody else must be creating them and that person was me.

CHAPTER 8 PLAYING WITH FIRE

At the end of September I decided, very anxiously indeed, to return to work when my current sick note expired. I'd been taking medication fairly regularly and I'd been bolstered by a quiet summer at home. I remember not actually thinking to warn anyone of my decision and just turning up on Monday morning, much to everyone's surprise. This just goes to show how inaccurate memories can be, as it is quite clear from the medical notes that preparations were made for my return. Sean discussed matters with my manager, telling her I was fit for 'light duties' only, and she is recorded as being 'quite supportive'. Perhaps my colleagues hadn't been told I was coming back and that's where my memory is confused. It was a Wednesday too, not a Monday.

I continued at work throughout autumn. My performance was mixed but at least nobody showed a desire to send me home, unfit. On a good note, I was responsible for realising an exhibition by a regional craft group. This was a relatively low-stress exhibition. There wasn't much creative input needed; it was more a case of working out how many display cases were required, making sure the information boards were correct and sundry other practical jobs. It may have been helpful that, as an exhibition, there was a clear deadline. To my surprise, and I think to my manager's surprise, I managed to deliver everything reasonably well. I was happy and relieved; it was the last positive memory I have of this job.

Unfortunately, I didn't really do anything else at work (or for that matter, at home). Most of my time was spent in the basement Art Store, where I would turn on the lights near the entrance, go to the back of the store and sit on the floor, in the dark, for hours. Sometimes, I brooded miserably about the goblins and the car crash that was my life. At other times I just sat, motionless, desperate to be at home and little more than a lump of breathing meat. At lunchtime, I usually ran home and then spent half an hour lying flat on my back in the draughty hall, stupefied. I can't remember why I ignored the settee; perhaps I was worried I'd fall asleep.

At work, back in that basement Art Store, I frequently thought about arson. Fire was beautiful and dramatic, and it would be a sort of glorious, grand end to everything, an affirmation of what I felt to be the goblins' great immeasurable power and magnificence. It was a vision that nobody else seemed to understand; they were too keen to reduce my problems to a mean, grubby, little illness.

Fire was also cleansing, the heat sterilising, so maybe it would fry the goblins and, if nothing else, convince the remaining ones to leave me alone. This was not an experiment I could try out at home. I was living in a terraced house, but the museum was a detached building with decent fire alarms, so I probably wouldn't kill anyone. There were plenty of flammable items down here in the basement; half of the store was filled with paintings, many of them oils on canvas. I was sure these would be easy to set alight, as they were drenched in turpentine. The goblins liked it in this basement so I would, no doubt, exterminate lots of them. Could fire purify the whole building? Or, even, the whole area? Would I be doing everyone a favour? But was it really a practical solution? Would the goblins be incinerated or would they just slip into the drains and appear somewhere else? They might appear solid but they were quite able to turn vaporous, if needed. Fairyland creatures generally can.

The goblins, unsurprisingly, were extremely enthusiastic at the prospect of a large conflagration and, in their familiar whole-hearted manner, it was the more the merrier when it came to fatalities. I was, as usual, deeply conflicted. After all, pleasing the goblins should be my ultimate ambition ... but why were they so keen on such irreversibly dangerous activities? It made satisfying them incredibly difficult. However, if I had wanted proof that arson would be a futile method of goblin removal, this was it. They were hardly going to espouse my fire-raising if it meant they'd be hurt.

There was also, thankfully, a further consideration lurking somewhere deep inside. The reasonable part of me had no illusions about the dangerous unpredictability of fire and the potential for loss of life. I liked and valued my colleagues; I knew all about their personal lives, and was fully able to appreciate them as people. I certainly wasn't setting out to murder anyone, however unintended, and I could only imagine with horror, the potentially devastating consequences of my plans. The goblins, as usual, with their love of one-dimensional ideas, never appeared to consider consequences at all. Should I really burn one of the finest buildings in the town and destroy millions of pounds of artwork and unique items of local history? The museum and its collections belonged to all the local residents and I was only one of them.

Overall, it was a poorly conceived plan, which didn't really go any further than the thoughts of starting the fire. As always, the goblins hadn't supplied me with a follow-up plan. They never did, being fond of grand announcements, and the detail was always down to me. What would I do after starting this fire? Would I escape? If I escaped, where would I go? Would I just pick up my possessions and go home, or would I join my colleagues at the fire assembly point, outside? Could I really stand there, a picture of innocence, knowing I was responsible? Or would I feel compelled to own up and enlarge upon my sensible justifications for this bizarre and dreadful deed?

More dramatically, would I mount the smoking ruins of the museum, with a flaming torch, shouting, 'Death to all goblins!' rather like the flag-waving maiden in Gericault's famous painting *Liberty Leading the People* - with evil goblins crunched underfoot, instead of dictators? I rather liked the last idea; I'd be a strong, responsible person taking on evil, but it was no more than a fantasy. I would never be brave enough. Anyway, my banner would more likely read, 'All hail the goblins!' and all that would be crushed underfoot would be millions of pounds worth of art and heritage, and perhaps a few of my unlucky colleagues.

Alternatively, I could stay and burn, a martyr to the goblin realms. If I were responsible for manufacturing the goblins - which I thought unlikely - then, theoretically, wouldn't my death fix the goblin problem? Truthfully, though, I wouldn't be brave enough to barbecue myself; cowardly me would, almost certainly, just run away. Then it would be back to the Broadmoor scenario, although, as I wouldn't be standing over a murdered infant this time, retribution might not be so inevitable.

Luckily, I didn't mention arson to my manager, which is probably just as well, as I don't think I'd have been allowed in the building if I had. I certainly wouldn't have let me in even though, in reality, I prudently left my matches at home. But the whole affair was deeply depressing to me. I couldn't understand why I was even considering such destruction. I was a museum curator; it was my job to look after precious things, not destroy them.

Yet again, things were being complicated by my inconsistent taking of the medication. In the early autumn, about the time I'd returned to work, I'd made some quite significant steps forward, as I had been taking medication fairly consistently under the supervision of the day hospital. For example, I'd started expressing a few doubts about the reality of the goblins, and even though there was an element of wishful thinking here, a hopeful 'positive mental attitude', I remember that there was some small substance to these assertions. This may have been partly because I was back at work, which had forced me out of the unhealthy loop of negative goblin thoughts, at least for some of the working day.

I also reported that goblins now only directly affected me and not other people. What a disputatious belief that had been. Nobody, absolutely nobody, had even countenanced this particular validation of goblin omnipotence. Of course, I'd provided a perfectly sensible explanation: they were being affected, they just didn't realise it. I didn't think people were stupid when they denied this control, it was simply that they were just unaware, and why would they be aware? Only megalomaniacs believe they understand more than the tiniest fraction of the world around us. After all, lots of nasty things happen to us all, so why couldn't they be the work of goblins? Other people blamed God or the Devil. They might be more culturally acceptable but were they, evidentially, more real?

Quite apart from ensuring I took medication, there had been a lot of input from Sean, over the summer and into the autumn. Looking at the medical notes, he was clearly persevering with the usual techniques: reframing, replacing negative ideas with positive ideas, explaining that it was just an illness, encouraging structured activity and all the rest. I seem to have generally gone along with this, although my attitude towards this input was very variable and, reading the notes it was, clearly, uphill work for both of us.

However, in autumn 2000, now back at work and with less professional support, my medication-taking became erratic and the brief window of opportunity was shut. It must have been deeply frustrating for everyone; I'd had so much supportive input. I was amply warned, by both Dr R and Sean, that any gains I'd made were not yet consolidated and, without medication, the goblins would reassert themselves. But here I was, as noted by Sean, on 18th October, refusing to take medication, yet again, and inevitably declining:

Jane now refers to her symptoms as the 'Goblins' again and stated it was wrong of her not to believe them and that she should not have got rid of them.

Antipsychotic medication ... Taking it, or not taking it, is a hugely controversial subject. In reality, most schizophrenics who go on to harm others are not taking medication; they've either not been diagnosed or they were, like me, medication non-compliant. I was very open about having command hallucinations to harm others, so it was obvious to mental health services that I was, potentially, very dangerous when unmedicated. It was probably my biggest risk factor, especially as it confirmed that I was unable to prioritise the real world (as enthusiastically promoted by mental health services) over my dangerous, unnavigable, internal world. It also showed my underlying personality to be impulsive and uncooperative, so difficult to manage. This toxic mix was compounded by my relative isolation: there were no immediate friends and family to monitor whether I was taking medication or not, or to keep an eye on my day to day behaviour.

There is a strong anti-medication movement, and if I'd stuck it out without medication I might, eventually, have stabilised. I would have had to have been in a very supportive environment to achieve this, but where would I get this support? At that point, nowhere, and it was nowhere again at a later date. There was never going to be a partner, supportive or otherwise and once my family were involved they were very clear about my need for medication. In fact, my mother once memorably told me that she'd disown me if I stopped medication again. I was also in conventional employment, so needed to be mentally stable, and amenable and useful, whatever was going on inside. It was proven time and time again that without medication, there was no way I could keep my thoughts on track for a whole working day.

It's difficult and painful for me to analyse my thinking at this time, but I have to remember that my challenging behaviours and beliefs were formulated in the murky, distorted world of paranoid schizophrenia. As a group, we are infamous for not taking the prescribed medication. I had all sorts of delusional justifications for medication non-compliance; these surface again and again in the notes, and I can't always assess the underlying motivations. Once medication was bound up in my delusional system, sensible outside arguments were totally undermined. Here are some explanations and justifications:

The goblins, for example, said I couldn't have medication,

probably as a punishment, and this belief was fuelled by a burning-hot well of hostility and fear inside me, complicated by plummeting self-esteem. At the time, at least by goblin standards, I believed that not taking medication was actually a relatively innocuous request, justified by my 'responsible' need to see what they were up to. It was a relatively easy way to placate them too. It didn't involve me murdering infants or attempting to commit arson on a grand scale. The only person it harmed was me. Was I aware that it was a form of self-harm at this stage? A nice, clean, tidy, blood-free act? Probably not; that realisation came later when I was less goblin-ridden.

I was, obviously, not able to think things through clearly but I'm not sure how aware I was of my intellectual limitations. Certainly, I didn't formulate a sensible plan for stopping the medication. If I had been realistic, it would have meant gradually reducing it over a long period. As usual, impatient me preferred an abrupt halt, rather in the same way one jumps into a cold swimming pool. 'One, two, three, it will be fine when you jump in, stop dithering ...' I only superficially accepted the inevitably unhappy outcome of not taking medication, even when the resulting damage to my mental health was painstakingly and repeatedly explained to me.

When it came to medication, everyone around me asked the same questions again and again. What's the problem? Just take the medication and get better. Where's the catch?

I'm writing this in 2021, during the great coronavirus vaccination programme. I've had my jabs, there's no way I'm an anti-vaxxer, as I'm more than capable of weighing up the pros and cons. People who choose not to have the vaccination I find mystifying and frustrating. Why wouldn't you accept something that saves the lives of the vulnerable, and unlocks the everyday pleasures of life for the majority? What's the problem? But then ... stop! Are they really so different from me? What right have I to be so critical of anti-vaxxers? Many live in relatively enclosed communities where misinformation is passed on by word of mouth and through targeted social media posts. Apart from the social media bit (effectively non-existent in 2000), this sounds suspiciously like my enclosed goblin world, except my community was even smaller, just me and the goblins really. Sensible and well-meaning outsider views, from whatever source, were tolerated by me, but usually no more than that.

I was consistently told by people that I had an illness. Illness? Possibly, sometimes, depending on who I was talking to. If you don't truly accept you're unwell, you're hardly going to accept side effects; sedation was the worst for me. A healthy, sane response to the situation would have been: 'I have an illness, it needs medication, the goblins are part of that illness, if I take medication the goblins will go (and stay) away, and I will get on with my life.'Frustratingly, with consistent mental health support, I nearly got there. Unfortunately, my rather unsophisticated counter-argument appears to have been: 'If I don't believe in goblins, then why am I taking medication? I'm well, aren't I? And medication is 'poison' anyway!' 'Poison' was a good catch-all description for anything I didn't like about it.

Then there was control, control, control. I was obsessed with flaming control. I appeared to have been a monomaniac on the subject. The word 'control' or sometimes, more broadly, the concept, appears time and time again in my medical notes throughout that autumn, as I announced that I had to stop the medication so I could take back control of my life - from both goblins and mental health services. I felt as though both were controlling me externally, twenty four hours a day; the goblins through their constant vigilance, and mental health services through the remote control of their unwanted medication.

I'm not saying this mental health service coercion was wrong, as I know my ability to function without medication was extremely limited. But I didn't have the insight to understand this, so mental health services had to take over my faulty executive processes. This was care rather than control, but it wasn't a distinction I understood in the least. Instead, I was extremely indignant when being harassed to take medication, and I felt infantilized by mental health services. Which in a sense I was. It's the only option when you've got a resistant patient with, at best, fluctuating insight; an insight that wasn't usually real either, as it was often just me regarding the problem as an outsider and not genuinely applying it to myself.

My care was, of necessity, reduced to simplistic statements. 'You have to take the medication otherwise you will be admitted to hospital.' Or, 'Take the medication, it relaxes the brain and helps you sleep.' Result: one ratty, disenfranchised toddler. I know, from experience, that toddlers, especially little girls, are extremely difficult to negotiate with when they misperceive themselves as responsible adults. In my defence, before my illness, I had been a functioning adult, perfectly able to run my own affairs. I'd had good jobs, looked after my money, kept my various homes tidy and all the rest. I was used to autonomy, if not at work, at least at home. It was very difficult to knowingly reinvent myself as a needy, childlike patient - however plausible a description when viewed from the outside.

Looking back, my medical progress of late summer and autumn turned out to be my undoing. As consistent medication enabled me to kick back at the goblins' control, at the same time I kicked back at mental health service's control - a control which was exemplified by medication. As the two were somewhat entangled in my head, it may even be that I thought freedom from mental health services - that is discharge as a non-medication-taking and healthy patient - would mean an automatic delisting from the goblin register. Then, if I didn't believe in goblins anymore, my freedom from mental health services should, I hoped, be imminent. These two concurrent views are totally inconsistent; it sounds like the chicken and egg conundrum. But to me, it would have been just 'win, win,' however that was achieved.

Most deeply, and instinctively of all, taking medication felt like a physical invasion of my body and, in particular, my mind, by mental health services. Hence it was obviously 'wrong' as unwanted invasions generally are. The goblins had invaded me and this, as everybody kept telling me, was wrong on all levels. Why, therefore, was an invasion by mental health services such a good thing? Their medication felt like an assault on my holistic perception of myself, and most of all my intellect. Surely, it was up to me to decide whether I needed something that was going to mess around with my brain? Not some random, however well-intentioned, outsiders.

Ultimately, medication non-compliance became a symbolic act for me, not that I realised this at all. It expressed my distress: look how I'm prepared to suffer to prove I'm in pain. I had no broken limb, nothing showing on an X-ray, no fever. It was all inside my head, so totally invisible. It expressed my emotional conflict, an emotional conflict I really didn't want. It expressed my rejection and a denial of an illness that didn't belong to me. And then what? What does a symbolic act really achieve? It might make you feel better but it doesn't fix anything.

Reviewing my medical notes, it was a confrontational autumn and although these conflicts were pretty low key, as my histrionics were internal rather than external, they do seem to have been pretty frequent. I took no pleasure in this war at all. I wasn't looking for attention and certainly not so much negative attention. It was awful being in conflict with everyone: it wasn't how I normally ran my life at all. I'm quite startled and embarrassed by how much input there was. Sean, the poor long suffering psychiatric nurse, was a model of patience and persistence. Sadly, I don't remember telling him that I was deeply ashamed by the amount of effort that was going into ensuring that I took the medication. I knew I was behaving like a distressed, delinquent child. I couldn't understand why I didn't just take the medication normally. What was my problem? Or, more pertinently, why did the goblins hate it so much? I had no idea. It wasn't even as though I liked not taking medication. True, it was sedating, but at the same time it made me feel better, both physically and mentally.

I'm all too aware that these paragraphs about medication don't add up to a coherent argument in the least. My views on medication, like my behaviour, were inconsistent and changed from day to day. There was simply too much going on for me to cope with - both acknowledged and unacknowledged by me. I wanted help from mental health services, especially as I was well enough to recognise that my life was disintegrating, while at the same time I was consistently rejecting much of the good advice they offered, effectively throwing their help back in their faces. Quite what did I think they could achieve on those terms? It looks as though I was expecting someone, somewhere, (or even me) to wave a magic wand and everything would miraculously right itself. Childish again, I guess.

Perhaps, going back to work was too ambitious and too stressful as, in retrospect, work seems to have been a goblin hotbed, but I was desperate to get back to a semblance of normal life. As a result, I slipped back into defensive patterns of behaviour; my usual 'touch me not' attitude. That's as close as I can get to my paradoxical, unhelpful behaviour.

Regular medication did resume, partly overseen by a support worker and also, as I can see from the notes, a few timely warnings about recourse to the Mental Health Act. I suspect that once that plan was being mooted again, I was probably more 'biddable'. About this time, Dr R, the regular psychiatrist moved on. I think I was sorry, but it's difficult to remember. She was a wasted opportunity, very conscientious and sincere and, if I'd been less intransigent, I'm sure she could have been helpful. Uncooperative, difficult me was now transferred to the consultant's list. The significance of this upgrade passed me by at the time.

The goblins seem to have welcomed this new player with their usual enthusiasm. On 1st December 2000, I was again refusing to take medication and informed Sean that this consultant, Dr C, 'was in league with the Devil'. I am talked round on the first point and take medication, but not, it appears, on the second. I have, for the record, no evidence that Dr C was anything but a dedicated and well-motivated clinician - certainly not a closet devil worshipper ... This sounds suspiciously like a goblin judgement, as goblins had a weakness for grandiose epithets and they were always keen to demonise people who were trying to help me.

CHAPTER 9 SUICIDE WOULD SOLVE EVERYTHING

During an autumn of inconsistent medication taking, I knew that my confidence was dwindling, particularly as I was aware, deep down, that had I taken the medication regularly I might have been able to reinforce my doubts about the reality of the goblins, and the validity and rationality of their ideas. Medication, medication, medication ... I gave myself no stability. Looking back, I was clearly trying to fight the illness, but only by blindly and persistently attacking my allies. It was a shame that all that energy, which was in itself a good thing, was so destructive. It could have been used for recovery. Instead, I effectively took hold of my life and chucked it in the bin. That's not a nice feeling, but you can't turn back time.

My low level, goblin appeasement continued. I didn't eat hot food at home for nearly two years, another goblin prohibition, and I was reduced to eating cold beans and tinned soup out of the can. Bang! It's one of those memories that lobs you back into the past; the smell and the look of cold baked beans is still stomach curdling, as they vividly recall the pain and desperation of that time. The cold food thing was ridiculous. I've never suffered from eating disorders so it was, presumably again, some kind of punishment. There was certainly no practical justification. When I'd moved in, I'd organised the replacement of the old lead piping for the gas supply and bought a cooker for the kitchen. This new cooker was to remain immaculate; not that the goblins objected to the cooker itself, it was hot food they banned.

Money wasn't an issue either, especially as my impoverished lifestyle was extremely economical. I could afford to pay gas bills. By the time I left the town, I had sore cracks at the side of my mouth and bleeding gums, both because of my low quality diet although plaque build-up probably contributed to the gum problems. (I didn't visit a dentist for years, even though I knew I had several decayed teeth). A bad diet is a causal factor in poor mental health, but I wasn't aware of this at the time, so it didn't occur to me that a lack of vitamins and minerals was hardly helping matters.

To be fair, as befitting their rather old-fashioned status, goblins showed no interest in modern technology and kitchen appliances whatsoever. I was never stopped from turning on the gas fires, for example, and they left the television and phone well alone. They confined themselves to announcing: 'You did that,' when there was something unpleasant on the television, but I regarded that as unwelcome goblin static rather than a genuine assessment of the situation. This was very good news; I was able to dismiss the accusation that I was responsible for the Twin Towers disaster the following year, amongst other things. If you ask me, 'What were you doing on 9/11?' I can tell you. I wasn't worrying about the loss of life, the terror of those trapped workers, the pain and bravery of their rescuers ... oh no. I was too busy telling goblins, 'It was really nothing to do with me.' It's been observed before: schizophrenia is an extremely self-centred disease.

As the nights drew in, and I became less and less useful at work, I brooded more and more on suicide. As I wouldn't, other than at a very superficial level, accept that medication could miraculously solve the issue of goblins, there was nowhere else for me to turn. Nobody could offer me any alternatives and neither could I think of any myself. So, what kind of independent future for me was there? I felt totally, hopelessly, overwhelmed. Wherever I looked, there was nothing but goblins and they appeared to be horribly permanent.

My soul, what was left of it, seemed terminally ill and my only designated future in the world was as a conduit of goblin evil. The more I worried about this evil, the larger, the more powerful, and the more complex it became. Hence the more terrifying. It also appeared, from my experiences so far, that I would never be totally possessed, and would never be unaware of my crimes. I'd always be cursed with the knowledge of what I was doing; a sort of helpless, sentient spectator, who'd be watching myself used as some kind of diabolical automaton. There was no relief, or hope of relief, at all. Was it even responsible to keep on living?

The following was written at work, in about mid-December 2001. It has photocopied museum catalogue information on the reverse of the page. It was in my medical notes, I think given to Sean so he knew exactly how I was feeling. I don't know how legible it was to mental health services, as it is the worst example of my handwriting I've ever seen. Not only is it a scrawl, but the writing is minuscule too. It's totally as written, except that I use the pseudonym 'Sean', for the psychiatric nurse.

We are all controlled by goblins. They have told us that we have reached the end, the end is nigh and everything will be destroyed, all eaten up. We have reached the end. No more. No more No more We are all controlled by goblins But goblins are a front - but for what? It's nameless and black and evil. There are layers beyond layers and layers upon layers The end The end.

I can't do this. I can't do this. I am all destroyed, all eaten up by goblins Goblins have destroyed my soul and destroyed my brain Everything is all destroyed Sean is my only hope and even he will eventually betray me Work is relevant to the main concern. I can't do this I can't continue pretending everything is OK. When it is not Beware the goblins, they are evil messengers They live all over the place and where people least expect them

My concentration is getting worse and worse I can't concentrate my mind is full of goblins and their evilness And as for the thing behind, the nameless thing How can I concentrate living with this knowledge I can't live with this knowledge It is too much too dark I must do as they say I must do as they say I must do as they say I must do as they say I must do as they say I must do as they say I must do as they say I must do as they say I must do as they say I must do as they say I must do as they say

Don't take medication I can see more clearly The medication blinds me to the truth, the reality of what is going on But if I don't take the medication they threaten me with hospital Hospital will answer nothing It doesn't get rid of them. They have goblins in their wardrobes They don't like me to take the medication because it makes me ignore them I have taken it for a few days That was wrong. I shouldn't have taken it I must tell Sean to go away This is what they say Tell him to go away. Tell Sean to go away. Tell Sean to go away. I must tell Sean to go away. I must tell Sean to go away I must tell Sean to go away I must tell Sean to go away I must tell Sean to go away I must tell Sean to go away I must tell Sean to go away I took the medication for the weekend CPNs, that was wrong I don't want to see Dr ... on Friday

I must do as the goblins say. They are messengers of the only truth Goblins are the messengers of the only truth Goblins are the messengers of the only truth

Kill yourself Kill yourself You must die to believe, that is the only way no taking the medication enables me to see the truth Medication hides the truth There is only one truth Medication hides the truth Medication hides the truth Medication hides the truth Medication hides the truth Medication hides the truth Medication hides the truth Medication hides the truth Medication hides the truth I must not take medication I must not take medication I must tell Sean to go away I must do as they say. I must do as they say I must do as they say I must not talk to Sean, he is too dangerous Cut him out - tell him to go away. When he says he is your friend don't believe him He is making up, he is not real He is a dead person come to tempt you to take medication Sean is not real Sean is not real Sean is not real But I don't want to go to hospital and if I don't take the medication they will put me in hospital. I don't want to go to hospital - they will make me take medication Medicine hides the truth Goblins are the messengers of the only truth Everything is falling apart. We are all controlled by goblins. We have reached the end There is no more We will all be

destroyed and eaten up by goblins. Goblins are the messengers of the greater thing that controls us all Goblins are the front. I can't work knowing what I know, there is no space on my head It is filled with goblins and their messages There are layers upon layers
If I see Sean he will out argue me and I will take the medication It is safer not to see him Tell him to go away Goblins, not Sean, hold the only truth. The truth is controlling.'

There's not a lot to add to this sorry piece as it speaks for itself. It really wasn't a good day at the office. I value its existence because I didn't keep diaries, so this is a rare self-authored account of what was going on in my head at the time. It's raw reading, proper madness. As much as I try to rationalise and explain my past, this is the truth. There's little trace here of my previously competent and educated brain.

The conflicts over medication come out very strongly, as illustrated by my contradictory attitude to poor Sean, who arbitrarily switches between a good cop and bad cop in my brain. My answer to this conundrum was to figuratively eliminate him altogether. 'Sean is not real' would have come as a big surprise to his family and friends, particularly as he was one of those people who appeared very warm and alive. I was desperate, deluded, paranoid, obsessive, confused and very, very frightened. No wonder I felt driven towards suicide.

In mid-December, I walked out of work at lunchtime vowing never to go back. My plan was to go home and kill myself, by hanging myself from a joist in the attic with a washing line - a washing line I had squirrelled away, especially for that purpose. My suicide seemed very appropriate, as I irregularly encountered the 'hanged man' on the landing of my house. This was what the house wanted.

'What the house wanted?' Since when had the house taken on a life of its own? The 'hanged man' had appeared intermittently since I'd moved in, and there was even a passing reference to him in my first encounter with Dr R, back in February 2000. He was not a victim of the goblins, so he appeared to be a separate problem. I had no idea why he was there. Was he some form of ghost? When he was in residence, always in the evening, I would take a deep breath when I went upstairs, close my eyes and scoot past. Otherwise, I couldn't get to the bathroom. 'Just go away please,' I'd mutter, feeling cold and unnerved.

Now, the reason for his presence was obvious. He was clearly a victim of the house, providing it with physical and mental energy. The house wanted more. It was showing me how to commit suicide and making it look easy. This, so-called hanging victim was as unmarked as a white candle; surely the victim of a strangulation hanging shouldn't look so pale and blank? He obviously hadn't suffered in death; neither, by implication, would I. This apparition, or whatever it was, was clearly some kind of visitor from the past, probably mid-twentieth century, as he had a short haircut, trousers with braces, and his shirt was not buttoned through. He would rotate gently, above a kicked away, wooden chair; in fact, crucially, it looked like one of mine - 1950s Ercol straight from my late grandmother's kitchen. So, there it was, a 'how to die' manual, carefully laid out in front of me. 'Look he can do it, he's brave enough. Now, it's your turn.'

I am not a great believer in the supernatural, basically because I've consciously experienced some of the human brain's nastier and more creative tricks. So, I'm guessing he was some kind of hallucination, especially as I recognised the chair, but there's always a small amount of doubt at the back of my brain. The house was old; what exactly had happened there? Was this hanged man some kind of replay, perhaps even totally meaningless? How many traces of other people were in the house, psychic or otherwise? Hair, skin flakes, exhaled breath, perspiration, blood, urine, semen, spit, breast milk, phlegm, wax ... all viscerally incorporated into the structure of the house.

Worst of all: thoughts. Millions of tiny thoughts milling about; did they feed the house? Was the house feeding on me? Were the goblins a feeding manifestation of the house? Were they no more than small, energy seekers, spiritually bonded into the house, as structural as the brickwork? After all, I had come to the house goblin-free. Yes, I already had the mysterious 'The Rules' - had they been hijacked and remade by the house goblins? Goblins who were just waiting for another dispensable, passing resident. That house was built more than a century before I was even born, and it's still there today ...

I sold the house in 2002, so I walked away from it both literally and metaphorically. It came up for sale quite recently and, for the first time, I saw the inside again, captured in the estate agent's photographs. What did I see? Essentially nothing; it was clean, tidy and entirely empty. In fact it had been noticeably improved by a subsequent owner. But I couldn't look at it dispassionately. Those neutral photographs were overlaid with an unspecific, lurid glow, a shape-shifting sense of dislocation; a moving image of red and purple worms writhing and boiling together, and a feeling of sulphurous heat. I clicked off the images quickly. Whatever's in that house I want no part of it. I don't want it realising my presence and emitting twisting, stinking tendrils to drag me back. Perhaps, however, I should be brave and return, knock on that familiar front door and offer to buy the house next time around. Then it'll let me, somehow, magically re-write my history.

No, I know the truth. There is no restorative magic. The house's sinister qualities are no more than my imagination, an imagination fired by my dark, angry emotions. Just in case, I've subsequently researched the house online. Had something terrible happened there? If it did, I couldn't find any reference to it.

After I'd walked out of work, that December afternoon back in 2000, my manager contacted Sean, my suicide plans were investigated and unravelled, and my washing line confiscated. I remember thinking these suicide plans were no big deal ... just another failure. Anyway, I was clearly preoccupied with much larger matters. Unfortunately for me, however, mental health services were unhappy about my nihilistic ambitions.

This is Sean, 14th December 2000:

> *Jane expressed that the end is near but no clear explanations as to what this was, but thought herself it meant that she had to kill herself. She stated she would be better off dead as she is no longer a person just a shell to do the goblins' bidding.*
> *I requested to accompany her to her O.P.A on the 15th Dec. Initially she was hesitant, said yes, then stated that she wasn't intending to go but would be now.*

I vaguely remember Sean taking me to the appointment and discussing Christmas arrangements on the way. I don't remember worrying about hospital admission. However, the fact that I was planning to skip the appointment must have meant I was suspicious. It was very unusual for me to miss a psychiatrist's appointment, however much I dreaded it. This was, though, a planned, and not an emergency appointment, and it had been agreed two weeks previously.

Dr C decided that I could not at the moment be safely managed at home, because of my increasing sense of hopelessness and the strength of my psychotic delusions. I was, unsurprisingly, 'reluctant' about admission so, yet again, the Mental Health Act was mentioned. 'This is all very unfair,' I thought. 'I'm more often than not taking the medication aren't I? And so what if I kill myself anyway?'

After the appointment with Dr C, I was taken home to pack some clothes. I was more with it this time and considerably better informed about what I'd need. Most importantly, I had to go home to break the news to my family that their eldest daughter was a certifiable lunatic. They'd been up to see the house, and I usually spoke to them about once a month on the phone, but they would be expecting me for Christmas and I couldn't see a way round this one. I could hardly say: 'I'm off to the Ecuadorian rainforest for an unspecified time, so I won't be contactable,' or that the hospital had an alternative line of business as a post restante. Poor mum, I remember her shocked, anxious voice. There are some things you really don't want to have to tell your family. After this sad duty, I obediently returned to the hospital. As always, 'go quietly' was my motto.

My admission interview report was somewhat more positive than last time. Thankfully, unlike the last admission, I was 'well-groomed in appropriate casual clothes.' I wouldn't consider myself a particularly clean or well-presented individual, but being admitted to hospital in 'dirty' (they weren't dirty as such, they were paint splattered) clothes last time had been dispiriting and embarrassing. Also, I was clearly more resigned to the whole admission process. For starters, I didn't inflict twenty five minutes of almost complete silence on my interviewer, and I do seem to have managed some rapport. Other than that, the interview comments are recognisably me. I am variously frightened and defensive, manage little eye contact, have reduced speech, flat affect, and express delusions of control and persecution, as well as passivity phenomena.

Surprisingly, for someone who was admitted after a failed suicide attempt, my mood was 'euthymic both subjectively and objectively'. Perhaps I should have cried, but I vaguely recall the interview in terms of a grey flat bleakness. I sound pretty bleak in the comments. My suicidal ambitions were ascribed to the strength of my psychotic phenomena. Once the psychosis was under control, everybody hoped I'd cheer up.

For the first time, I now had positive family involvement from both my parents and my aunt. This was both a relief to me and especially to mental health services, who had for a long time fretted about my relative isolation (in both senses of the word). This meant I got to go home for Christmas. My parents drove the 200 miles to rescue me. I remember seeing them standing at the end of the ward, near the guarded door and looking totally out of place. They represented 'home,' didn't they? Certainly not 'prison'. It was as though a photograph of them had been superimposed on the ward, like some kind of hallucination. But they were, thankfully, real enough. They were also prepared to take on a lot of responsibility. I wasn't aware of this, but letting me leave the ward with them for Christmas was not something Dr C wanted to do. They looked pretty shell-shocked after he interviewed them, without me, and they told me that if I caused them any concern whatsoever I could be delivered back at any time of the day or night. Rather like Battersea Dogs Home. On a plus note, that interview meant I didn't have a lot of explaining to do, which was a relief.

I don't recall much else, including any details of that Christmas. I presumably took medication and made no suicide threats, and was returned to the hospital by my parents as agreed. In spite of the distance, I wouldn't have been allowed to use public transport, which would have made it easier for them. It's pretty obvious that mental health services were effectively in loco parentis, which was a nasty surprise to all of us. I was my family's problem, wasn't I? My family were no more aware of the legalities of mental illness than I'd been at first. Nobody in my family had ever been admitted to a psychiatric ward, and while there was, inevitably, some mental illness amongst my relatives, nobody else had achieved such a spectacular implosion. Even though I was, at least on the surface, somewhat more resigned to the situation, in truth I was still in a state of horrified disbelief about the whole affair.

On the ward, I would apparently smile at staff when approached but otherwise communicated in monosyllables, and spent all my time sitting on the bed in my curtained cubicle. In other words, I was mentally attempting to 'not be there' (in mind if not in body), while remaining semi-alert to the obvious dangers of my immediate environment. It wasn't a very successful combination, but it was my usual way of coping with the stresses of the place. I would, however, away from the oppressive, noticing, incarcerating atmosphere of the ward, talk to anyone who'd take me out into blissful fresh air, even if it was a slightly forced conversation. I wanted such rescuers to know how much I appreciated it, basically so they kept rescuing me, and it was easier for me to talk outside, as I was no longer choked by the ward environment.

The only other memory I can dredge up is of catching a bad cold from someone on the ward and feeling very cross about this, reasoning, probably correctly, that had I not been forced into hospital, I would have remained cold-free. My priorities were clearly all over the place, as I seem to have found my cold far more bothersome than my serious mental illness and suicidal feelings.

As I found the ward such a hostile environment, it also looked as though I was taking refuge in the goblins. Perhaps, somewhat desperately, they were a preferred loco parentis for me (certainly preferable to mental health services) especially as my own parents had returned home. After spending Christmas with my family, it sounds as though I was feeling lonely and somewhat lost. On 4th January 2001, Dr C noted about the goblins:

> *She finds them 'supportive' and 'nice' at times, despite their instructions to harm herself. "If I kill myself I will be with them."*

By mid-January I was considered generally improved, and was discharged home with compulsory attendance at the day hospital. I'd now learnt that if you wanted to avoid the psychiatric ward you had to a) take your medication b) not make suicide threats c) attend day hospital as required and, finally d) if threatened with the Mental Health Act, amend behaviour immediately so the subject is dropped. With these points in mind, I was confident I wouldn't be admitted again.

After the December admission, I didn't return to work. The next two months can best be described as bleak and, even with the help of my medical notes which I'm relying on quite a bit for structure, I remember very little. I seem to have been regularly attending the day hospital, where I did various arts and crafts with two jolly, occupational therapy ladies. I didn't want to be at the day hospital, where I felt horribly self-conscious and monitored, but if I was going to have to be there, making a cushion cover was a tolerable activity. I've still got it and periodically wonder if I should throw it away, since it's loaded with unhappy memories. However, I can't quite bring myself to do so, as I can't believe the extreme neatness of my piping. Bizarre. I'm sure I've never managed such competent sewing before or since. What else was I doing? All I can recall are hazy impressions and feelings.

The goblins, having sucked all the life out of me, had the same effect on my environment. The townscape looked like so many grey cardboard cut-outs, as though I was in an old- fashioned photograph. Of course, there must have been other humans about, but they seemed lifeless and inaccessible to me. Certainly, not much of a challenge to the goblins. The only bright points were mothers with babies in pushchairs. I don't mean bright as in joyous, I mean the sickly brightness of a thermal imaging camera. I always slid my eyes away from the babies as soon as possible, as this was the only way I could protect them from my damaging gaze. It was all deeply shaming and painful, and those babies burned both my retina and my brain: goblins never allowed me to forget. On 29th January 2001, Dr C noted:

Feels hopeless, depressed, Goblins also derogatory "You are useless and cannot manage without us."

In February, there was a medication change to another atypical antipsychotic, risperidone. 1st March 2001, Dr C noted:

Infanticidal thoughts present again. Speaks of a 'mission' to suffocate her friend's baby because it is evil. Sees this partly as irrational but urged by goblins. In her imagination sees herself gaining access to her friend's house innocently and then taking her opportunity.

Dr C telephoned my unfortunate friend; she was, apparently, still 'keen' to continue the friendship. There are times in life when you can only marvel about how kind people are. She was prepared to keep knowing me even though I was prepared to destroy something infinitely more precious than me: her baby.

By 15th March, I had been refusing risperidone for the last five days as it caused me anxiety. This, I do remember well, as it made me extremely uncomfortable physically. I was otherwise willing to take medication - anything to stay out of hospital - and I agreed to take the previously prescribed medication. Unfortunately, and predictably, my mental health had deteriorated during the last few medication-free days. The goblin hit list appeared to be expanding. Dr C noted:

> *Goblins telling her to thrust kitchen knife into 'Sean' CPN (she has told him), and to throw any passing baby under a bus. So far it has not been too difficult for her to resist.*

That was probably just as well, on both counts. I'd moved on from figuratively erasing Sean, to actively (in principle) erasing him. He had, by now, wisely transferred our meetings to the back room, where there was a kitchen table between us, but he continued to visit me alone. Brave man. I guess that Sean probably thought that I wouldn't attack him, and he was right; I was horrified by the nastiness and violence of this goblin ambition. Yet again, I was having sordid, nasty, dirty thoughts and they made me feel very unclean. However, Sean was an ex-member of the territorial army and a strong well-set-up individual, so he probably thought that if things had got sticky he would have been able to disarm me. For the record, my knives never made it out of the kitchen drawer when he visited. I wasn't even tempted by this particular goblin instruction, so his brave assessment of me as 'basically harmless' was, in this particular case, correct.

I clearly had ambivalent feelings about Sean, as evidenced by the goblin hostility. The goblins, quite correctly, saw him as a threat to their dominance, especially as I liked, and usually trusted him. He diligently challenged them every time we met, extremely patiently, even though it was a very repetitive task; in other words, boring. It was this persistence that landed him on the goblin hit list. I did listen to him, and he was able sometimes to moderate my belief system. However, he was also an agent of the evil mental health services which were not loved by me, and even less so by the goblins. Hence, he was, in my eyes, fundamentally compromised.

Unfortunately, by 19th March I was back to my usual behaviour and, in another appointment with Dr C, making a fuss yet again about taking medication, because, 'I was not ill,' and, 'didn't need it.' Oh dear. I suspect that by the 15th, I'd been off the risperidone for too long to be clear-sighted enough to realise that medication non-compliance was not a wise decision. I had also been refusing to attend the day hospital; in other words, I was breaking the sensible 'How to stay out of hospital' rules I had enumerated to myself only in January. I was described by Dr C as, 'tense,' and at times, 'clearly very preoccupied,' but later said that I would take the medication. This was probably because I'd suddenly realised that another hospital admission was looking imminent. The only bit of the 19th's conversation I vaguely recall was:

Dr C: 'I think it would be a good idea if you came and spent some time on the ward with us.' (Psychiatrists are good at non-confrontational phraseology.)

My response? Along the lines of, 'I don't think it's a good idea at all. Why do I have to come in? I said I'd take the medication, didn't I?'

As usual, mention of the Mental Health Act soon resolved that argument (it was a piece of legislation I was, by now, heartily fed up with, as it seemed to have been invented to persecute unfortunate people like me). I agreed to be admitted as a, so-called, voluntary patient. Apparently, I would benefit from a medication change under supervision. Unsurprisingly, I took a very dim view of this as, in spite of everyone's reassurances, I couldn't see that the goblin problem was at all fixable, so was not at all keen to be locked up for an indefinite period of time. It was, I reasoned, patently futile and totally unfair, as even a prisoner knows the length of their sentence. That all this might be for my own good, as ever, totally passed me by.

I was obviously still angry during the admission interview with another junior doctor (no 'rapport' established), later that day. He wrote:

> *Thought content: difficult to explore as guarded & not really forthcoming. No evidence of delusional ideation, no FTD, no passivity phenomena, no obsessional phenomena ...*
> *Denies suicidal id. Denies intentions of hurting others at present ...*
> *IMP DD between Psychotic Dis & Psychopathic personality.*

Quite frankly, it sounds as though I would have denied my address, if given half a chance. It's probably as well that I didn't read this until recently, as it is another object lesson in 'How not to speak to psychiatrists.' My bad-tempered reserve presented as psychopathy. That said, I am very grateful to Dr C, who added to this description: 'Re above - I do not think she has a psychopathic personality, however that term is defined.' That's a relief. Goodness knows what kind of havoc I could have caused, if the admitting doctor's assessment of me had been correct.

CHAPTER 10 HOPE

It was back to the ward. When I arrived, having trailed home and packed (described as having 'run off' after the appointment, so slight difference of opinion there), the nursing staff said, 'Hello Jane!' brightly. 'Oh great,' I thought, 'everybody here knows me now.' Being known by the local psychiatric ward's nursing staff was definitely not one of my life's ambitions.

It was also back to the same ward routine and, for me, back to my routine ward behaviour. As described in my medical notes: preoccupied, self-isolating, guarded, avoiding eye contact, usually pleasant if approached, but no more. In other words, my attempt to be a good, quiet girl who could be released forthwith. As ever, it never occurred to me that my good, quiet, rational and reasonable behaviour was totally invalidated by my obsessive elucidation of the baroquely nasty goblin world. In addition, sitting on my bed doing absolutely nothing for hours, day in, day out, on a sort of semi-alert, watchful, standby mode like a rabbit in a trap, hardly showed a desire to engage healthily with real life, especially as I apparently refused to attempt the small amount of occupational therapy on offer. What exactly was I doing or thinking? Mostly, I can't remember, so my guess would be nothing, nothing at all.

As a result of my overall quietness, there was very little drama in my hospital stays. I was never forcibly restrained or forcibly injected with medication but, quiet or not, inpatient stays were hardly restful; they were a physical and mental ordeal. I don't think the nursing staff were aware of how I felt; I just presented as 'withdrawn' or 'aloof'; these terms appear again and again in my notes. My only private space was a curtained cubicle in a dormitory and I spent most of my time there, so I didn't have to speak or interact with anyone (bar goblins). I felt safest at night when I could hide under the bedclothes, much as I did at home, but here, on the ward, getting up and staying up was supervised. Every morning, I sat quietly (up and dressed) and listened to the less tractable patients versus the nursing staff, engaged in the 'it's time to get up' war.

Nurses described my communication with the other staff and patients as monosyllabic or superficial. 'What's the point of me talking to any of them?' I thought at the time. 'How can talking alleviate my problems?' I could talk about goblins, all day long if required, in a rather circuitous and extremely repetitive manner, but how could flimsy speech have any effect on powerful, menacing goblins? It was hardly going to disempower them. Meaningful conversation, I believed, was as pointless as tackling a war armed only with a toothpick. Why bother, when it was such hard work and in such an alien environment?

Of course, I was supposed to bother during the weekly ward round interviews, which seemed to involve a cast of thousands including, memorably, a visiting doctor who fell asleep. However, I was apparently so intimidated by ward rounds that Dr C took to talking to me individually. He was right, I did speak more openly when there were just the two of us, as even I had realised that he was the bloke with all the power, and my best route out of hospital was to exert myself and offer some preferably reassuring insights into my mental state.

Looking back, my most painful memories of hospital were almost exclusively regarding various deprivations of liberty. I was still hugely, massively resentful about this. Why wouldn't I be? Breaks from the 'dangerous' ward represented the only relative safety I could access. Certainly, in the nursing notes, I was generally mentally inaccessible except when somebody tried to take away my small freedoms and I would become agitated and, very occasionally, tearful. Any idea that these hospital coercions were for my own safety entirely passed me by. I wasn't interested in my own safety or, to be honest, the safety of others, even if other people were.

By now, on my third ward admission, the world outside was an obsession. I spent hours looking out of the window, charting the ebb and flow of hospital life. Then there were the ordinary homes, barely visible, beyond the hospital walls. I'd have given anything to be living in one, especially when their evening lights went on and I imagined everyday routines - evening meal, television, privacy, autonomy, normality and most of all, safety. Although, even I had to admit, this utopian view of other people's lives would be somewhat moderated by reality.

I also gazed wistfully at my bed sheets. These were sometimes woven with the names of other hospitals, presumably the result of some central laundry cock-ups. Perhaps, if I were living in one of these other areas, say Southend, my life would be totally different, and a free and entirely sane me would be happily walking along a beach; a sort of magic carpet to a more palatable existence. Hmm. Really?

The ward had no enclosed outside space at all, so I could only get fresh air by standing right by a hospital window which, of course, only opened a crack. Thus, physical freedom, however limited, was my be all and end all. When accompanied outside I was extremely conversational just so there was no doubt that I was massively thankful, and, please take me out again. Anybody? I think I would have happily gone out with Attila the Hun, if he'd been the only 'patient walker' on offer. It was such a physical and mental relief not to be on the ward.

A community psychiatric nurse (Sean was on holiday) very kindly came and took me out two days running, immediately after my admission. We walked about in wet snow and had basically normal conversation. I remember it so clearly; I was hugely grateful. She must have found the contrast strange as, a week earlier, she and another nurse had come to my house and I'd apparently refused to speak to them, other than minimally, and had asked them to leave. In passing, I barely remember my impolite and hostile treatment of these well meaning, visiting psychiatric nurses. Embarrassingly, however, it's recorded again and again in my notes.

Ward staff only had time for a fifteen minute march to the front of the hospital and back. This task usually devolved to a student nurse. I remember one who was obsessed with lighthouse maintenance; his previous, obviously much regretted, job lost to automation. 'Oh help,' I thought. 'How am I going to say anything pertinent about modern lighthouses?' I knew all about Grace Darling and J.M.W. Turner, but they were hardly relevant. Luckily, my reputation for being mostly silent was well established and I wasn't expected to say anything much at all. We always ended up at the hospital helipad, just in case the air ambulance arrived. It never did. 'When I was a lighthouse engineer, we used to take helicopters to the more remote lighthouses,' he explained, wistfully. I don't know how he went on as a psychiatric nurse but I learnt a lot about lighthouses. This, somewhat one-sided social exchange on my part, was probably categorised as 'superficial'.

My parents and aunt were my most regular rescuers, but it wasn't easy for anybody as my parents lived so far away. My aunt, who was closer, had a round trip of ninety miles but I was so relieved to see her, I didn't really consider that. Occasionally, we drove out to the countryside and I recall a great deal of laughter (an extremely rare occurrence at that time) when I was nearly swallowed alive by the mud at Knott End. When we were at home, she would sit by my front window overlooking the street so she could keep an eye on her Porsche. It was not the usual kind of car for the square and the infrequent passers-by liked to inspect it. I was always glad to be home, so I could have a bath and do my washing. I think there were washing machines on the ward but, as ever, I was too shy to ask. There was only one bath (each dormitory had a shower, but I don't like showers) but the water was always lukewarm.

My unaccompanied leave from the ward built up gradually and I treasured it, as it was the only time I felt relatively alone and free. It was hardly exciting; initially it was limited to a daily hour in the hospital grounds. It was a large, general hospital, so 'grounds' with its implication of stately house grandeur, is an optimistic description of a reality that was mostly concrete with some scant greenery around the perimeter. My favourite spot was a dismal, rectangular concrete pond with an even more dismal islet in the middle. That spring, the pond was visited by a duck and her ducklings, and I gazed at them fondly, while considering the depth of the water, whether anyone would be looking out of the nearby windows, and whether I could, therefore, drown myself. I didn't mention these unhappy ideas to anyone, so nobody banned me from visiting the pond.

At this point, when alone, anywhere outside the hospital was forbidden, thus extremely alluring to me - even the very dull, local streets, which I occasionally visited out of boredom, and the chance to gaze at something that was less redolent of my incarcerated status. Then someone spotted me, and I was taken aside and reprimanded. Yes, reprimanded and warned - my unaccompanied leave was a privilege, not a right - for setting foot on a quiet, suburban road. This was a stark reminder of my peculiar situation; I was, after all, an officially informal, voluntary patient. I wasn't under section but, even so, the ward staff had an enormous amount of power to regulate my life. Perhaps Dr C, or the nurses, thought I might be tempted to run away, as I could hardly get up to any mischief in those forbidden streets, the goblins having no particular hostility, or even views, when it came to tidy 1960s homes and their admirably neat gardens.

As any potential curtailment of liberty upset me deeply and I would do anything to avoid it. For several weeks the new medication, clozapine, gave me low blood pressure throughout the morning which I was desperate to hide, in case I wasn't allowed to leave the ward or, even worse, have my admission extended. But, there were a few times when I couldn't hide it and I remember, for example, very briefly fainting in the morning medication queue. I couldn't dodge that one, as I was hardly inspecting the ward's flooring and, yes, my ward leave was suspended.

I was interviewed and examined by a junior doctor about this episode, but I don't seem to have offered any useful insights into the problem, even though I knew, perfectly well, it was probably low blood pressure. It didn't occur to me that I was being unhelpful and, as a result, the ward staff were left to work through the options. So, I had an ECG (normal except for sinus tachycardia which was probably stress-related); what I ate was monitored (normal but sometimes pulled up for skipping breakfast, which was actually because I felt too dizzy to stay upright, but wasn't going to let on); and then they finally settled on low blood pressure. This could be objectively measured without any input from me at all, except for sticking out my arm.

Unsurprisingly, I continued to avoid speaking to my fellow patients but I watched them closely (mostly so I could avoid them, just in case someone wanted to talk to me; to be fair, they didn't - even the very chatty ones soon gave upon me) and observed that many of them had very brief admissions indeed. I was amazed when Sean informed me that there were people who liked being on the ward - that is, cared for - and would even come to A&E on a Friday night, so they could be admitted as emergency cases and not be properly assessed until Monday. You what? This was clearly madness. As far as I could see, if you were desperate to preserve your liberty, like me, you were thrown into hospital, whereas if you were begging to be admitted to the hospital, you were turned away. Maybe my approach had been wrong all along? Or, perhaps, it was more a question of insight.

Ward security was ever-present and difficult to forget. The front door to the ward was kept locked, I think by way of a two way keypad. Certainly, the access number was limited to staff. The police were regular visitors and, consequently, great friends with the nurses. I covertly watched unfortunate people being delivered to the ward by the police, and the police taking descriptions of escaped patients. The only escape I could allow myself was thinking enviously of these brave runaways. I wish ... I wish ... I gave no thought at all to their individual stories and how they subsequently managed.

I obsessively fantasised about running away. For some reason, I was fixated by Hull. No idea why, other than that nobody would ever look for me there, and it was an inexpensive part of the country. I hadn't even visited the place, well, not properly; my sole experience of Hull was a brief glimpse from a minibus window, on the way home from the ferry terminal. It had looked pretty bleak at 7am on a wet Sunday several years ago. Perhaps, my selection was instinctive, as it fitted in well with my prevailing mood at the time.

However, I didn't act on these fantasies and nobody knew about them, as I'd been well and truly scared by Sean's warnings about what happened to voluntary patients, but those liable for sectioning, when they absconded from psychiatric wards. He assured me that if I bolted home the police would come after me and, if they suspected I was there, and not answering the door, they could force entry. I found this a very alarming thought indeed. How would I get the front door fixed? Would I be asking ward staff for the numbers of joiners and locksmiths, and trying to arrange things from the ward payphone? I imagined my house with a missing front door and all the local low-life squatting in my front room, destroying my possessions. As intended, it was all deeply daunting, so I didn't run away, however great the temptation.

So there we are. Paradoxically, I had built a belief system for myself that was all about curtailing my freedom. Anybody listening to my account of what the goblins made me do, or wanted me to do, would think I was desperate to live in a totalitarian state. The ward should have been ideal. I can only guess that the more the goblins controlled me mentally, the more I treasured my physical freedom. It was my chief escape route from the unhappiness and frustration of my life. Walking is well known to bring bodily and mental relief, and the long view was comforting after the forensically detailed, goblin claustrophobia. I also took comfort from the sight of people going about their daily business. I didn't know them and watching them was, generally, emotionally peaceful - unless they had pushchairs, which complicated matters.

Back at the hospital, I was definitely improving. The goblins still chaperoned me constantly, particularly hanging round the cubicle curtains or, apparently, in hospital wardrobes. I don't remember this last assertion but it's in my notes, and it's possible the goblins were seeking out the kind of dark secluded space I would have liked too. To be honest, I would have loved to have achieved total invisibility: 'I'm on your stupid ward, as required, you just can't see me!' However, I could hardly spend my days in a wardrobe as, never mind attempting to act normal, everybody would think I'd absconded. Yet again, I suspected that the goblins were not entirely sure how to work around all these new externally-imposed hospital rules, so their actual activity levels were low. They were used to having me to themselves.

However, the goblins cheered up when I left the ward by myself, and especially when I was eventually allowed to get the bus home, by myself, each afternoon. The bus stop was by the kind of scrubby woodland strip they particularly liked, so they were usually hanging about there, waiting for me. I wasn't too bothered by this because it was the kind of low level interference I was used to. I never thought how, eighteen months ago, in my less troubled pre-goblin existence, I might have viewed this peculiar situation. The goblins chitter chattered about suicide, but I was so glad to see home that when I actually got there, they were reasonably quiet.

In June, after about three months, I was discharged, with compulsory attendance at the day hospital yet again. Dr C had wanted me to stay as an inpatient for longer, but dear, kind, altogether lovely Sean had told me I was no longer sectionable anymore, so there was absolutely no way I was going to stay a second longer on the ward than I had to. Objectively speaking, my ward existence was healthier than my home life, but that didn't worry me in the least.

The medication change had been to clozapine, which is recommended for treatment-resistant schizophrenia, and is usually initiated in hospital because of side effects. It did seem to be working; there was overall much less goblin activity and their instructions were less violent too. When my employer's occupational health department asked for a report on me, Dr C wrote that I might be able to return to work, if not immediately. I was cautiously optimistic about this as well, especially after discharge and through July. It was a frightening prospect but I did feel more positive and overall less distracted. Perhaps, I wouldn't after all have to destroy my everyday life - relinquish my house, give up my job and all the rest. It would be just as well, as there wasn't an alternative plan.

At home, I more or less drifted but, under duress from mental health services, signed up for some charity voluntary work. I assiduously attended my pre-arranged sessions, steaming second hand clothes (a tedious, but safe activity) and being on the till at another shop. This was more exciting but felt extremely unsafe. It didn't occur to me to say that I didn't want this stress; I'd had the usual supermarket checkout girl experience in the past, so I was reasonably competent. I also went to the day hospital as required where I actually, according to the notes made about me in creative classes, seem to have been reasonably well engaged and even mildly friendly. Discussing goblins, one to one, was never something I enjoyed but being required to make a coiled clay pot was a relatively low-stress activity. Other than that, my life was essentially blank. I spent a lot of time in bed, fully dressed, doing nothing, and watched a little television. It was quiet at home, especially when the school children were on holiday. When there were funerals at the church across the road I got to hear the muffled passing bell. It was a spooky sound.

Yes, I did see a few old friends and family, but other than that I was living in a state of total spiritual poverty. My every day, escapist pleasures were inaccessible to me. I didn't, for example, read a book for three years, and I had no interest in art and art galleries. Art and antiques are in my lifeblood and I remember being encouraged to visit an art gallery, so I took the train to Liverpool, to visit the Walker. It was a pointless excursion; I couldn't engage with the art at all. It was totally meaningless;

never mind lack of concentration, my head felt totally empty. I've had a deeper emotional and intellectual response to the council bin day leaflet. After a few minutes, I turned around and went home.

Would things have eventually righted themselves on clozapine? I'll never know. In August, my white blood cell count dropped too low - a recognised, potentially dangerous side effect - so I had to stop the clozapine for good and wait for my blood counts to stabilise before I could be started on another antipsychotic. For the first time, I was being told not to take antipsychotic medicine, just when I had been taking clozapine, regularly, as prescribed. The irony of the situation didn't escape me.

Predictably, things started to slide quickly in spite of the non-antipsychotic medications, such as the sleeping pill, temazepam, which were prescribed to keep me going.17th August 2001, telephone call, community mental health team, 9pm:

> *Refused to take px Temazepam stating she was "training to be a goblin and goblins don't sleep." Also disclosed that after her training she would kill herself so that she would be a goblin - did not know when the training would finish.'*

I settled down once antipsychotic medication was prescribed again, but the fragile gains of the summer were lost. My last window in the town had closed and, for the first time, it wasn't my fault.

CHAPTER 11 TOWARDS AN END

The final six months of my life in the town were little more than a dreary blur. The goblins continued to be troublesome, but I can't see any new issues in the medical notes. As ever, my insight seems to have varied and, as usual, there are some positive comments.

29th October 2001, psychiatrist letter:

> *Jane is a little more settled though her passivity phenomenon remain. She has also gained a margin of insight in that "the goblins sometimes tell lies because their threats do not always materialise."*

I was never able to sustain these breakthroughs. This particular step forward wasn't firmly entrenched as, a few weeks later, there was a minor break-in at my house which, unsurprisingly really, had little to do with the town's low-life and more to do with goblin punishments. I don't seem to have been asked how I thought that this might work. Was the house breaker directed to my house by goblins? Was the house breaker actually a goblin? I expect if I had been asked, I'd have managed to come up with some form of explanation. I generally did and if not, I'd just say: 'I don't know. The goblins don't tell me everything.' While thinking: 'How am I expected to know everything about goblin activities and their obscure reasonings?'

Just in case there were any doubts about goblin omnipotence, I also announced, on several occasions, that they were responsible for 9/11 (previously, the goblins had blamed me for 9/11, but I seemed to have forgotten that refinement). Goblin interference could be guilty of bathos; while not destroying large buildings and killing thousands, they were, apparently, prime suspects for supplying a dodgy, meat pie that gave

Sean food poisoning. I remember Sean's imperfectly concealed frustration when I told him this, but I couldn't understand his negative reaction. It was a perfectly reasonable explanation wasn't it? It didn't occur to me that he'd been seeing me for more than eighteen months and we were still stuck; I was still, arrogantly but unconsciously, forcing my delusional world on to other people's lives.

I was still obsessed with burning down the museum. When asked about the potential loss of life, I told the psychiatrist that the victims 'wouldn't mind,' as they'd become goblins. Lucky them. But I showed myself fully aware that whatever the victims, or rather their loved ones, thought of this somewhat surprising outcome, nobody would be at all grateful and I'd end up in a secure hospital. It was the same old story. Other people's rights? Whatever. My own liberty? Vitally important. Naturally.

The consultant, Dr C, moved on and I was downgraded to an older doctor, Dr H, who was perfectly pleasant but seemed a little deaf. This downgrade was good news. I hadn't managed to kill anyone, so I was presumably considered less worrisome, although on 13th December 2001, Dr H described me as 'still undeniably a risk'. I wasn't used to having to speak up when it came to goblin explanations so it was an odd feeling; speaking more loudly is something you do when you want to emphasise veracity. As I was perfectly aware nobody wanted me to ascribe any veracity to the goblins at all, I was used to outlining their activities quietly.

So, there were differing degrees of 'same old same old', except my spirits were sinking lower and lower as I realised I'd spent two years dismantling my life. Yes, I had a lot to show for it: unfortunately, none of it was positive. I had no idea how I was going to get back to a normal lifestyle, as I seemed to be becoming increasingly institutionalised. In desperation, I asked to go back to work on a voluntary basis, especially as my employer's occupational health department was again enquiring about my mental health. Their consultant in occupational health interviewed me. The following is taken from his letter to my psychiatrist, Dr H, dated 22 November 2001:

> *It sounds as though she has quite a resistant schizophrenia and when I saw her this afternoon, she was clearly not very well ...*
> *One of the reasons for her wanting to get back to work apart from the obvious normal ones was to find out what the goblins were up to in the Art Store ...*
> *I would ... specifically be interested on your views on a voluntary basis ... and whether you think it would be reasonable to expect her to be able to get back to a job involving contact with the general public, planning and arranging displays and really quite high level performance.*

I am, quite frankly, amazed that the occupational health doctor even considered my request. What did he make of the goblin bit? He sounds dryly amused; it can't have been a usual argument for returning to work, particularly when mixed in with, 'all the obvious normal ones'. I do remember talking to someone in an office during this period, possibly him, and beseeching them to let me return to work so I could monitor the goblins' behaviour, as it really was essential that somebody did ... but I'm guessing it wasn't this time, as no comment is made on my delivery, calm or otherwise.

Dr H's response to this letter was a very cautious 'Yes' to a possible part-time return in March 2002 but, as both the occupational health consultant and Dr H noted, this would be challenging as work was a hotbed of delusional goblin activity. Unsurprisingly, voluntary work turned out not to be an option. My suggestion raised all sorts of practical issues that had not occurred to me. What about insurance? Was I sick or not sick? Would I need to be constantly supervised? More fundamentally, was it just prolonging the inevitable? Rather like trying to salvage a pot plant with only two sickly small leaves. I was also the employment version of a hospital bed-blocker; my post at the museum couldn't be filled until I'd finally resigned.

On one level this was a disappointment, as I saw it as a route back to normal life, but then again, was it really true that I could achieve meaningful voluntary work (i.e. not sitting in the Art Store doing nothing)? Or was it something I believed *I ought* to be doing; the familiar toxic script, which had got me into this mess in the first place. I could kid Dr H and the occupational health consultant but I couldn't kid myself. There'd be an emotional and/or goblin uprising - the exact details depending on your perspective, but catastrophic in both cases.

Perhaps the introduction of goblins in the occupational health interview was an unconscious desire to sabotage our meeting. Or maybe it was a way of expressing unmanageable emotions as, for all my brave talk, returning to work terrified me. My last working memories, from almost exactly a year ago, were of total dissolution and despair. It was hardly a safe environment for me, especially the gothically reimagined Art Store. My heart still contracts with fear as I envisage it now. The low light, barely penetrating a smoggy charcoal darkness, the tomb-like frigid dampness, the slow drip ... drip ... drip ... somewhere, just out of sight - quite apart from the seething, termite-like, evil goblins.

No, that's totally ridiculous, of course it wasn't like that. It was warm, dry and well-lit, just as you'd expect for a secure area housing valuable artworks. You wouldn't even know you were in a basement, apart from the lack of windows and the number of service pipes. And was the problem really the Art Store? What about my wrecked concentration, motivation, self-confidence and, more generally speaking, brain? There was no way I could achieve 'really quite high level performance.' So, I don't think this refusal of voluntary work made much difference to my working life.

After the clozapine failure, I was prescribed older antipsychotics; haloperidol (I refused to take this as it made me anxious), thioridazine (stopped, not by me, because of possible cardiac side effects after ECG), and then back to sulpiride.

After I'd jibbed at the haloperidol, I settled down to medication compliance.

Finally.

I'd had enough of unscheduled admissions to hospital and lengthy discussions on the subject of why I needed medication. All that correctly worthy persuasion eventually wore me out. I had no energy to fight anymore. I wasn't exactly in agreement that medication was a good idea, but I'd eventually accepted that not taking it was a bad idea - not just for me, but for everyone around me. Lukewarm, I guess.

Unfortunately, my previous history of medication non-compliance was amply recorded in my notes. When, after Christmas that year, I was more unwell than I'd been for a while, it was recorded on several occasions that my current medication compliance was 'debatable'. This view must have been confirmed by a risk assessment handover sheet with the 'uncooperative' box ticked. It was odd reading this some years later, as I'm usually quite a law-abiding, conscientious person who avoids rows, although I can be somewhat contrary. Anyway, it was a good cautionary tale that served me right; that if I were unwell it could be ascribed to me not taking medication and not, more accurately this time, because I was just, well, ill. Not that I thought I was particularly ill, in spite of overwhelming evidence to the contrary. At least I was consistent, if that's a virtue.

I don't remember having much to say at all to mental health services, unless pushed. My threats to hurt people meant I was quizzed incessantly on the same subject and I always ran out of things to say. For two years, I'd been having conversations with people about goblin violence and **I still didn't understand why they found the subject so fascinating and alarming.** I put this last bit in bold ... as it's so telling; it demonstrates a total lack of insight, a total inability to empathise and a total degree of self-preoccupation. That's what schizophrenia is. The ultimate bad, bad ego trip.

My loss of will to fight anymore, so good in terms of taking medication, was a clear indicator of my spirits. My mood, during this period, was described in the medical notes as low, but not low enough to warrant medical intervention. I remember complaining, regularly, that, 'the goblins had stolen my words,' which was sort of true. Thanks to the illness and/or goblins, my life was impoverished and so was I. No concentration, no interests, no ambitions, no life. So, of course there was nothing to say about it. My head felt almost totally empty. I could virtually hear a prairie wind blowing through it, and what little brain I had left was splattered against the inside of my skull. As far as I was concerned, the goblins had cleared me out. It was pointless trying to help me, as there was nothing to build on, nothing to recover from, nothing to encourage or nurture, nothing to value or love or even like. There was nothing left.

Just after Christmas 2001, Sean moved on. It upset me profoundly, as I was very reliant, probably over-reliant, on his input. I don't believe I made a big deal of it externally; however I felt inside, partly because of the circumstances. He'd actually been seeing me for a while, strictly unofficially, as he'd moved to a different service. How he'd arranged this I'm not sure, but I really appreciated it. I don't know if I ever thanked him properly, and I don't even know if he was paid or not during the last months. Selfish me never thought to ask.

Sean was a very kind, patient and optimistic individual. There were times when he must have been deeply frustrated and bored (I would have been), as we went over the same ground endlessly, but he was careful not to show it - well, mostly; he wasn't a saint. The cold, nasty, dried-up goblins, with whom I spent so much time, contrasted strongly with this warm, pulsating living being. It gave me so much relief when I was with him. Sean was naturally amusing, which in those last few sad months I treasured. We'd trail through the usual goblin litany of misery and varying degrees of potential violence, then he'd tell me the ups and downs of his domestic life and it always gave me some relief, albeit fleeting. Occasionally, I saw him at the day hospital and I always knew if he was already there because I could hear all the staff laughing. Unlike the other nurses, I almost never told him to go away.

He'd never shown much anxiety, and always asked me to be honest, even though he had to listen to me saying some very alarming things. There are details in my notes about the possible involvement of forensic services, but this referral wasn't made, as it was felt I would find it too upsetting. In spite of the threats the goblins had made against Sean - or rather the threats I had made - he'd continued to visit me alone. The goblins really didn't like or trust him one little bit. Throughout that autumn of 2001, my medical notes record me saying on several occasions that I needed to, 'get him before he got me'.

I'd actually mostly trusted Sean, although I was always unreasonably fed up when he reported back to whichever psychiatrist was managing my care. I used to ask him,

'Why did you tell Dr ... that?'

He'd look at me seriously and reply, 'I'm a nurse, Jane, it's what I do.'

It was a strange relationship. To win my trust, which had been challenging, he'd behaved like a friend, but, of course, he wasn't a friend at all in the true sense. We wouldn't even have met otherwise, quite apart from becoming friends, as we came from totally different worlds and we were incredibly different people. Most importantly of all, he was being paid to talk to me and luckily I never forgot that.

However, had Sean been a manipulative psychopath, who enjoyed counting his conquests, I was there for the taking. If he'd have said, 'Run away with me!' I would have run after him with barely a moment's consideration, even though I fully realised we'd be a disastrous match. I was a vulnerable, needy, lonely young woman, and he was a good-looking and kind, slightly older man. It certainly didn't occur to me at the time that my feelings of love, or perhaps more my fervent desire for emotional support, were only inspired by one aspect of his overall personality - the one he brought to work - and that I was effectively re-making him to suit me. That said, I didn't worship him. I was more than capable of assessing his character failings, or rather what I identified as his character failings. When it comes to these, he would probably beg to differ.

Thankfully, for both our sakes, I was also perfectly aware of boundaries, quite apart from the unavoidable fact that he was well out of my league. I certainly made no attempts whatsoever to attract him; I remained an under-washed, crashing bore. Fortunately, my illness never took the form of erotomania; I was usually frightened of people rather than chasing after them. Overall, there was no way I was going to jeopardise my relationship with Sean; I valued him too much. But I want to be honest about the situation; it's the dark side of the therapeutic relationship. As I'm writing this, I can imagine Sean choking on his beer with horror at the very idea of life with me, and it makes me laugh. I can't look any sillier than I do already. Psychosis is a great leveller.

Poor Sean. He'd given so much and there was so little to show for it, at least on the surface, but he had made a difference: all that practical help was locked away inside me, but it was there nonetheless, waiting for when I could approach things more objectively. Even at the most basic level, he'd never abandoned me, thereby consistently challenging my theory that anybody who knew about evil me and the goblins could possibly think there was anything worth salvaging. So, the psychiatric nurse I had so hostilely rejected at the beginning of my involvement with mental health services turned out to be the most positive memory of my whole unhappy journey.

Had I not had such a good psychiatric nurse, would the thoughts have been worse? Could I really have killed someone? As I'd never had consistently regular support from other members of the team, I couldn't make comparisons so, at the time, I didn't appreciate how lucky I'd been.

Now, my closest confidant on the subject of goblins had gone and it also coincided with me finally leaving my job. My medical notes go from dreary stability before Christmas to dreary instability in the New Year. I was increasingly upset, and Dr H noted that, 'as usual any mention of goblins distressed her.' I can't remember how, or when, I'd gone from my usual flat repetition of goblin affairs to this distress, but I was obviously feeling very pressured by practical matters; I was all too aware that things were coming to a head after I'd spent the previous year drifting.

All this emotion was painful and unmanageable and it had nowhere to go. The 'distress', noted by the psychiatrist, was a cul de sac emotion; I didn't open up and discuss why I was distressed, which might have been helpful. I just shut down the conversation. There was no crying, or shouting, or becoming angry, but it's clearly expressed in what I baldly announced, for example noted on 6th February 2002, by the home treatment team:

> *When asked what would happen to her if she could not return to work "I'll have to become a goblin" - confirmed this meant she would have to kill herself.*

I remember sitting with a very nice nurse who was completing a care plan, and having to resist very powerful goblin instructions to snatch the paperwork from her, scribble all over it, tear it up, and then possibly jump on it, followed by me hitting something (not, fortunately, the nurse). This was presumably so I could release the pain, but I didn't fully realise this at the time. I mostly, but not entirely, thought that it was the goblins who'd decided this particular piece of paper was such a bad idea. I can't remember quite why the goblins themselves were so against it; possibly the nurse was asking too many questions and I felt threatened. As for me? It was just more unwanted form-filling and assessments; there had been so many, all futile.

This can only have been the recent, more distressed me, because a potent desire to destroy someone else's carefully completed paperwork was a new feeling, which is why I remember it. I suspect that there was a certain amount of wishful thinking going on here and that somewhere, deep down, I hoped that destroying the paperwork would somehow help destroy the goblins. Writing things down about them was always at this stage a talismanic act, an unsafe thing to do. Thankfully, even I could dimly perceive that it would be neither a polite or helpful way to behave.

Sadly, none of this emotional turmoil showed on the outside, so I got no help with it. Here's the nurse's account of that meeting, on 5th of February 2002:

> *Jane attended Home Treatment this morning, she presented as very quiet with little or no eye contact. I introduced myself as her keyworker ... which she seemed disinterested in. We discussed her care plan and she re-read and agreed to ...*

It's difficult to imagine that this is an account of the same meeting.

Those last few weeks in the town, involved another outbreak of paper about me, and my suicide threats, lack of self-care and all the other sad indicators of a malfunctioning life. If I'd been brave enough I would have killed myself, no question, but, as usual, I couldn't overcome my fear of death. It wasn't being dead that worried me; I had no belief in any form of afterlife and death was just an unequivocal full stop. It was the process of getting there that frightened me. I'd be sure to mess it up, and what if I changed my mind halfway through?

In my ideal world, mental health services would have relieved me of the responsibility for orchestrating a successful suicide and quietly finished me off; the equivalent of sending a car to the scrapyard. My spare parts, i.e. organs, could then have been recycled and distributed amongst more deserving human beings, but murder, however deserving the victim, really wasn't part of their job description.

I seem to have had a lot of input from both the home treatment team and the day hospital: a whole procession of well-meaning strangers were, yet again, crashing about in my world, monitoring and organising my life. Possible hospital admission was mentioned in the notes, but I probably avoided this setback because, in spite of people's doubts, I was medication compliant. I vaguely remember all this unwanted attention but not, as it is recorded in the medical notes, that the day hospital was compulsory and if I didn't go I would be tracked down and threatened with readmission to the ward. This was, as ever, a very effective warning.

During this period I spent increasing time with my parents, where I was both mentally and physically fitter than I was when alone at home. Once I'd resigned from my job, they decided it was time I was permanently rescued and brought back to live with the family. I can't remember - I was so preoccupied with losing my job - exactly what I thought about this, though yet again my inner conflicts come out in what I said. 21st February 2002, day hospital nursing notes:

> *We talked about how the Goblins had not took Jane's parents into consideration and how she has their continued support for the future, she said she was worried that the Goblins would have some influence on her parents health, maybe a stroke or a heart attack.*

Was I really worried the goblins would damage my parents? Or was I just saying that
I shouldn't be allowed their help? Either way, my parents' health stayed intact although some years later my mother died of a stroke while my father survived a heart attack. I really do believe that this was coincidental and that the goblins had nothing to do with it.

As far as my parents were concerned, the northern town's mental health services had reached the end of what they could do for me. It had been two years since my initial referral, and unfortunately, through no fault of mental health services, I was in a worse state than when we'd first met. I'd taken two years of medical support and then what? The give and take nature of therapy had been a closed book to me. I genuinely didn't understand how it worked. I'd given a certain amount, just enough to string people along, and then much of what I'd taken I'd rejected and thrown back. In my defence, I was so out of touch with reality that I hadn't even realised I was doing it and therefore effectively torturing myself by prolonging my individual version of hell. So, my internal goblin life remained largely unmoderated and, for me, soul destroying.

I was now in the limitless wastelands of chronic schizophrenia.

PART 2

CHAPTER 12 FAIRYLAND

If this was a fictional horror story - which is what I intended when I first started writing this - then the supernatural would probably be the dominant theme. I was going to trade in the goblins for something less bizarre and unintentionally humorous, though I hadn't worked out quite what, and I was going to develop the haunted house theme more fully. I was also going to link it into the 'idea' of the city as a living organism, posited by Le Corbusier amongst others.

Then, I was going to mix in some non-supernatural madness of the 'will she, won't she' variety. My favourite novel on this dilemma is Patrick Hamilton's incredibly atmospheric *Hangover Square* of 1941, but there was no way I could come close to matching this. I read a lot of fiction, and I carefully and objectively examine all fictional books on madness. While I accept that everyone's experience of madness is unique there are, perhaps, some rather suspect creations out there. You could argue that fiction is just that, fiction, a creative process disassociated from reality, so anything and everything is valid. However, I know from my own reading that fictional worlds do shape our experience of the real world; so in some ways they function in the same way as non-fiction.

After a great deal of consideration, I decided to stick to the only honest horror I know: my own story. This, unfortunately from a plot point of view, doesn't feature any real dead bodies - even if it is gorily littered with metaphorical ones. It's also distinctly repetitive, but that's the whole point when it comes to elucidating my obsessional form of madness.

My account is, I hope, a balance to some of the more lurid non-fiction found in the popular press; well, about murder, usually. It's been said many times before that the psychotically mad tend not to murder solely as a result of their madness.

Unfortunately, though, that's not always the case, which is why the most bloodthirsty of my command hallucinations were taken seriously. Many psychotically deranged murderers have other substances in their body at the time of the crime - usually illegal drugs or quantities of alcohol - but I never did.

I particularly wanted to show how easy it is to get from functional normality to dangerously deranged without involving any psychoactive substances whatsoever. Accounts of psychosis go back centuries and most of its sufferers have been as drug and alcohol free as me. But in recent years many, many accounts of psychosis, written by patients and/or loved ones, involve cannabis or other illegal drugs and/or excess alcohol. These are often vivid and moving stories, and I would, in no way, want to diminish their validity and their need to be told. However, I do wonder if these stories risk inadvertently rewriting the psychosis story in the minds of the general public, tainting every psychotic story with the suggestion that illegal drugs or too much alcohol might have been involved.

Cannabis, in particular, can trigger psychosis in vulnerable individuals. The word *trigger* is the key here; sadly, some of these patients would never have become psychotic without some degree of substance abuse. It can tip the balance in an already vulnerable brain. Humans, to my deep frustration, don't come with an operator's manual (my manual should have included the red alert warning: 'Don't get too stressed!') so there's no way, currently, of identifying people who are best off, like me, avoiding anything stronger than weak coffee.

As is clear from my account, I am not one of nature's risk takers. Although I wholeheartedly adopted totally irrational goblins, I'm not an open minded thinker, be it justifiably or foolishly depending on your viewpoint. I've got the wrong kind of brain; the bits I'm aware of are very prosaic. Who knows about the bits I'm not aware of ... I wouldn't go so far as to say that religious beliefs, of whatever colour, emanate from the unconscious brain. I'm well and truly out of my depth here, but it does look as though my 'religious' beliefs (i.e. goblins) must have come from my unconscious brain.

My everyday brain had absolutely no idea what to do about this sudden outbreak of 'faith', so I approached the goblin problem with a very narrow point of view. If I had sought out and been more open to other interpretations of the problem, perhaps the outcome might have been different. In particular, I might have discovered some relief amongst like-minded people. But my thinking was incredibly rigid; I believed in goblins and nothing else, nothing else at all.

Therefore, I was not remotely interested in exploring further theories and would close down any tentative discussions on the matter. This was partly because my belief in goblins didn't make me at all accepting of the reality of other fairyland creatures. If somebody implied that I must believe in will-o'-the-wisps, giants or, most especially, gnomes (yep, still writing about that one through gritted teeth), I considered it insulting. I was a grown-up, wasn't I? It never occurred to me that to an outside observer, logically speaking, why wouldn't I believe in other phantoms?

Those outsiders, who were trying to keep track of my internal world, had only my guarantee that we were sticking with goblins. It was a pretty worthless guarantee too, considering that my grasp of reality was fatally compromised. I was extremely defensive when outsiders pointed out to me that there were numerous, goblin-type things of no apparent interest to me whatsoever. Why was this the case? Why was I just limiting myself to goblins? (Possibly, or possibly not, backed up by the Devil, depending on my state of mind.) I didn't realise that they were worthily trying to chip away at my newly and unhappily acquired goblin mythology. I thought they were attacking me.

As far as I was concerned, my adult belief system was totally intact (skipping over the controversial issue of goblins) and I was keen to keep it that way. This meant it was essential that no other random peculiarities were given any air time at all

... just in case. The 'just in case' was my underlying protective position. I really believed the goblins would never go away. I did, however, have some underlying anxieties that they might be joined by goodness knows what else, which may or may not be bubbling away in my psyche or, even worse, hanging around on the lookout for an unwary host, i.e. me. After all, goblins had made the leap from storybooks so who, or what, else could? What other horrors were out there eying me up? Limiting my party to 'goblins only', gave me an illusory sense of some control over the amorphous, uncontrollable and generally unreasonable supernatural world. Or, perhaps, the amorphous, uncontrollable and generally unreasonable real world.

That said, of course I was fully aware of the huge pressure from the outside world, a world in which outsiders demanded I should jettison my belief in goblins. As a result, listening to goblins usually felt wrong, a dirty compulsion that I shouldn't indulge in. I made no efforts to back up goblin belief through research; I don't remember at any stage visiting the folklore section of the library to find out more about them. My feelings were very mixed. On the one hand, I would have considered it a very dangerous act indeed, while on the other hand, as a just about functioning adult it made me feel what? Disobedient? Ashamed? Disapproved of? When I worked in a local charity shop, I would shy away from any book at all that mentioned the word goblin in the title, or even if I thought the book, whatever its title, might have been infiltrated by a stray goblin or two. For whatever age group. Yes, I really could be frightened of books aimed at the under sevens. 'Know your enemy' is a useful tool when it comes to containing fear but I refused to even countenance the idea, so the goblins' all-encompassing, evil magnificence went unchallenged by me.

But, I didn't invent goblins, however they manifested themselves. The next paragraphs are a basic list of places where goblins or goblin-like creatures can be found. There is a strong psychological basis to the concept of goblins. They and their friends have been used for centuries, in various different cultures, to explain the distressingly inexplicable and general anomalies of life. This is clearly how I used them. I was farming out anxiety, anger and all the rest but, at the time, I was totally blind to this obvious explanation.

It is difficult to study traditional art history, as I did at university, without learning quite a lot about the Bible, the Apocrypha and the histories of saints. St Anthony, for example, was tormented by some very strange beings indeed. I'd also had a conventionally Christian education in both primary and secondary school. In passing, goblins themselves don't feature that much in standard art history, but some of the 'things' that populate Breughel's visions of hell and other doomsday type representations are not dissimilar. In Biblical terms, goblins probably come under the banner of evil spirits which may, or may not, infest the unwary. Was I infested? Well, yes. Did I look to God and the Bible for relief? No, it didn't even occur to me. I was totally convinced from day one that the goblins, as wayward creatures of the natural world, had nothing to do with religion, organised or otherwise. It also never occurred to me that religions of the natural world, such as paganism, would be at all relevant. I didn't seek spiritual help at any stage.

I was, however, broadly aware of ideas of exorcism and possession, but casting out unclean spirits, religious or otherwise, never crossed my mind. I was also aware of suggestions that unwanted spirits can infest vacant or damaged souls. I suppose you could argue that suppressing my emotions had left a void which the goblins could fill, but I wouldn't necessarily see this as a supernatural problem. Initially, I believed the goblins were raiders; ideas of possession came later, when I believed I was turning into a goblin, but I didn't see this as a possession that could be exorcised. It was more a spiritual and bodily evolution.

The finer points of 'demonic possession' were totally unknown to me, but I do want to acknowledge them here, as I know there are sad cases, sometimes even tragic, when people believe that a mental illness, which could be helped by medication, is actually a manifestation of hostile, supernatural forces. Importantly, my own 'demonic' (or goblin) possession was, more or less, successfully moderated by antipsychotic medication.

Demonic possession is usually divided into four stages: identification, oppression, possession and death. They vary a bit depending on what you read or which television programme you watch; there is a phenomenal number of television programmes, both fictional and documentary, dealing with the subject. I could argue that I picked up a demon infestation in the first flat in the northern town (the first appearance of 'The Rules') and had taken it with me to the new house, where it manifested itself as goblins. Goblins are, supposedly, a helpmeet of the Devil. I was certainly oppressed and, later, sort of possessed, but then? I'm emphatically not dead, even metaphorically speaking. I suppose it's possible that the demon still lurks within me, like a poisonous cluster of cancer cells waiting to spring back to life ... but this really is an unhealthy enquiry. If I follow it through, I risk scaring myself into my past.

Persevering, however, I do sometimes find long scratches on my body when I wake up. Some people say that these can be inflicted by aggressively evil spirits during the hours of darkness but I've noticed, as far as I'm concerned, that they occur during times of stress and are probably self-inflicted, as are various other night-time irregularities. (How did the battery get out of the clock again?) As a child, I occasionally sleep-walked and regularly talked in my sleep too, so I'm used to the idea that sleepers can carry out actions forgotten by morning. Any goblin bed-shaking - this happened periodically - can be ascribed to hypnagogic hallucinations, rather than a gang of hooligan goblins enjoying a night out. *Fungus the Bogeyman*, first published in 1977, and written and illustrated by the extraordinarily talented Raymond Briggs, now comes to mind. It's hugely entertaining, as well as being essential reading for anyone bothered by things that go bump in the night.

However, sceptical as I am, I can't really be one hundred percent sure my problems are entirely medical, so my research into demonic matters has been superficial and doesn't include anything other than reading and a small amount of television. Those awful supernatural 'reality' television programmes are as effective as demon possession anyway. They really can sap the will to live, as they effectively take our destinies out of our hands and sacrifice them to powerful and unreasonable malevolent beings. Like goblins really, so I know how disempowering and depressing that feels and how fundamentally dangerous it is as well. Anyway, I have never sought out real-life priests, crosses, Latin incantations and practitioners of purification rituals (sage is best kept for cooking - I am allowed to cook these days). Just in case.

There are various other interfaces between supernatural theories and madness. For example, strong, repressed emotion can, at least theoretically, cause or contribute to poltergeist disturbances. Or there's the stone tape theory; my 'hanged man' could be an example, his image embedded in the fabric of the house. The list goes on. I certainly hadn't investigated these paranormal ideas before my illness, although I was, like most of us, mildly curious. The only 'real life' ghost story book I'd read, prior to my goblin infestation, was a Harry Price book on Borley Rectory, at one time immortalised as the most haunted house in England. I'd been quite excited when I started to read it, hopeful of some general enlightenment or at least curiosity-provoking ideas, but it was actually rather dull and not very convincing, so I gave the book to a charity shop. In fact, I now read far more ghost stories, both real life and fictional. I find them comforting, as the people in them have a far worse time than me and their problems can't be fixed by pills. Importantly, though, I'm not convinced that these stories are true. Possibly, possibly not. It's quite fun reading them, although, as far as I'm concerned, madness is much more terrifying, so I won't be returning to Harry Price any time soon.

I certainly had not (and have not since), in any shape or

form, experimented with other aspects of the occult. I'd never so much as touched a deck of tarot cards or a Ouija board; never knowingly visited a haunted house; and I'd never drawn a chalk pentangle in a disused church prior to sacrificing a goat … at midnight. Continuing on, I didn't have a background belief in New Age theories. I'd never given much thought to astral projection, the Bermuda triangle or past lives. I'm not saying these ideas are wrong, it's just that I'd always had no more than a passing curiosity in them. Crystals, especially the large ones, can be awe-inspiringly beautiful and potent reminders of the earth movements that made them, but I didn't, and still don't, believe they could fix my mental health, toothache or anything else.

Within living memory, my ancestry was devoid of soothsayers, fortune tellers and faith healers. Not even a rumour or a half-remembered story. There were no artists, poets or any other obviously creative people in my lineage either. In fact, my relations had distinctly functional jobs, such as building and engineering. I didn't sit at either grandmother's knee in an old family farmhouse listening to traditional tales of fairies, brownies, imps, elves and, of course, goblins. One grandmother died when I was very young and the other liked urban life: Du Maurier cigarettes, Aristoc stockings, and frozen peas. No gothic fantasies here. My grandparents' home was a nice, un-haunted 1930s detached house in south Manchester, though it did have a turret for the stairs. In passing, my parents' home was a nice, un-haunted 1920s detached house in the home counties. My mother looked wistfully at houses with a turret for the stairs.

There are, of course, the officially fictional goblins. Yes, I'd read Christina Rossetti's classic poem *Goblin Market*, but it wasn't something that had made much of an impression on me. I'd also studied Shakespeare's *The Tempest* for A-level, which does feature some secondary, magical goblins, but I can't see how they were ever more than a passing reference in my brain. I was totally unaware of the Green Goblin supervillain in Marvel comics. Reading through the Wikipedia discussion of the Green Goblin's history, I can't see any links to my own life at all, and depictions of this Green Goblin are totally unlike mine. Going back further, I did enjoy fairy tales as a child; maybe I was scared by a goblin - they never come out of these tales well. As said previously, my goblins look most like the drawings of Arthur Rackham, so that's the best I can do with this line of enquiry.

Whether I liked it or not, I was being controlled by officially supernatural beings and I've still no real idea where they actually came from. I can look at it from every angle and admit that you can't rationally explain away a goblin. They are just not culturally valid in 21st century Britain. Over the last century or so, the only little green men in the ascendancy have been aliens. My inner world seems to have been impervious to these more up-to-date manifestations. If I were a believer in alien phenomena in their various forms, this could have been an extra-terrestrial story, but I've never so much as knowingly glimpsed a possible UFO. However, the northern county I was living in does have quite a record when it comes to UFO sightings; then again, it's a large, well populated county.

After all these considerations, I've largely (but not conclusively) given up on the supernatural, in all its various guises, in favour of science. This was, in part, helped by intriguing books such as Richard Wiseman's *Paranormality,* (2011) in which the author explores how so-called supernatural experiences provide vital insights into the intricate day to day working of the brain.

Unsurprisingly, I'm very interested in how the brain works, and more especially how it misfires. How did I go from a normally functioning person to, well, a total nutcase? There's been a lot of fascinating and amazing research in the last twenty years into the inner workings of the brain, some of it the result of PET scanning which allows researchers to see the brain functioning in real time. I was going to try and summarise it for this book, but there are so many different studies out there that I found it too complicated. The traditional medical summary is roughly this: the psychotic brain produces too much dopamine;

this excessive dopamine makes it difficult for the brain to manage external stimuli successfully; therefore the brain struggles to create a serviceable understanding of the outside world. The main treatment, antipsychotic medication, works by blocking or partially blocking various dopamine receptors in the brain. Different antipsychotic medications target different patterns of dopamine receptors.

Any more complicated than that and I was straight down the rabbit hole, and into the mysterious land of rat studies. Not that the newspaper headlines mention the rats, this particular qualification tends to be embedded in the main text. Then there are other studies, which, for example, identify possibly significant abnormalities in the Zq2ABTgxC neural pathways ... Yep, totally lost (in the interests of scientific exploration, I made up this pathway). My entire science background is an 'O' Level in biology, a very long time ago. I can't remember what this involved, other than inspecting algae growth on tree trunks and an odd visit to the swampy school pond.

Certainly, strange things lurk in one's genes. My father, enthusiastically tracking down our mostly mundane forebears, has had my DNA analysed; I've chosen not to pay for the medical analysis as I'd really rather not know more than the basics. In spite of the Englishness of my recent ancestors, I appear to have inherited a lot of Irish genes and it has been anecdotally observed, and now scientifically proven, that rates of psychosis are higher than average in some parts of Ireland. These are driven, at least partly, by certain genetic mutations. The particular genetic mutations may have been triggered by the Irish potato famine - and yes, my ancestry does include the sort of poor agricultural labourers who would have suffered greatly at this time. These mutations, presumably, increase the risk of responding badly to adverse life experiences.

There's also, unsurprisingly from my surname, some Highland Scots. Both the Irish and Highland Scots have a traditional, and rather impolite, reputation of being 'off with the fairies'. Well, I can't argue with that, as I appear to be living proof of this description of psychosis, so maybe I'm some sort of genetic throwback. While I would have crossly repudiated the idea that I was having trouble with leprechauns, I am aware that they are a subset of goblins. Thank goodness I wasn't controlled by leprechauns, as they're possibly even more embarrassing than goblins. My goblins had neutral English accents anyway.

Then there's the sixth sense. This has been used to describe various innate human skills, such as the ability to locate one's body in space, to use echolocation, and possibly to tap into the earth's magnetic field. What else is this sixth sense capable of? Can it pick up on other-worldly creatures such as goblins? Could goblins in fact be real? Or are they 'real' in a parallel universe? In non-linear time? To be honest, almost certainly no, but where do you draw the line? When does a scientifically plausible reaction segue into a hallucination? Who defines it? It's all very murky.

Overall, I've learnt from reading books and articles that the human brain is capable of getting up to all sorts of mischief, much of it totally unknown to, or unexamined by, the bit we call self. Goodness knows what's going on in the neural borderlands. Our brains are hard-wired to look for patterns and explanations constantly, so it can process the mass of information coming in from outside. We make mistakes all the time and they can usually be dismissed. Perhaps the goblins were originally some kind of mistake in my perceptions - possibly no more significant than that.

So, in trying to look for the cultural, autobiographical or supernatural source of the goblins, have I actually been chasing after shadows? Were the specifics of goblins just incidental? Were my goblins triggered initially by accidental readings of light and shade in foliage? Did the cracks in the plaster of the house suggest a nasty little face? Were goblin voices no more, at the beginning, than the creaks and pops of an elderly, not very well-maintained house? Was I making spoken external commands out of white noise? Was the whole 'selection' of goblins I've spent so much time analysing, no more than a trick of the light? Or a trick of the ear? Was it no more than that I had an overload of negative emotions which needed to be hung somewhere - anywhere but me - and the goblins were an accidental hook? How many other negative beings did I come up with and dismiss, without giving them a second thought? Did the goblin pattern occur randomly, several times, and was eventually embedded in my brain as reality? Were my goblins were no more than a bunch of visual and auditory triggers, jammed together and given form by me? And did it, perhaps, have something to do with the name of my new vacuum cleaner - Goblin?

CHAPTER 13 DELUSIONAL ARCHITECTURE

Or how to maintain your delusional world in spite of overwhelming evidence that you might just be wrong …

A private psychologist, Dr A, once told me that to support my goblin world I made up explanations as I went along. He wasn't suggesting that I was consciously creating the goblins for some obscure reason of my own, it was more that I refused to examine them properly and recognise that they might, just possibly, not be real. Either way, I was highly offended by this accusation (or helpful remark depending on where you're standing), as I took it to mean that I was deliberately creating inadmissible excuses for the reality of my goblin metropolis; in other words, that I was deliberately confabulating.

'How could this be correct?' I thought. I was sure that I was basically truthful. If you wanted to catch the liars, then chase after the goblins, not me. Of course, he was right, but I was doing it largely unconsciously, even though my delusional world was not a happy place to be. I was in a permanent state of inner conflict, as I tried to balance the demands of my internal and the external world (or the demands of my unconscious and conscious world). When I look back at goblindom, it is a mass of half-explained, half-realised contradictions. My delusional construct was supported by lies throughout. This is an exploration of some of these lies, lies that I only learnt to address with hindsight. How could I address these lies at the time? As far as I was concerned, the actual structure and workings of the goblin world had precisely nothing to do with me. I was manipulated, managed and bullied by goblins, but it was one way traffic. Nothing I said, or did, or questioned or believed, would have any effect on the goblins whatsoever. That was obvious wasn't it? Why couldn't outsiders understand this?

When supporting your delusional world, there's one very simple foundation statement: 'I'm not ill'. Everything else is built on this. If you want to get better, you have to embrace your illness, however profoundly you detest it. It was many years before I just about accepted this deeply unpalatable truth, and, my God, it improved matters. It was the end of best foot forward, and compromised acceptance: 'I might be a bit ill … at least while you're standing in front of me making me take medication, or interviewing me in hospital, or trying to make me feel better about goblins,' and all the rest. How I managed to stick to the idea that I was not ill when presented with various psychiatric nurses, psychiatrists and enforced admissions to hospital, I have no idea, but it's a well-known and troublesome aspect of schizophrenia and complicates treatment in many cases, not just mine. Obviously, I didn't feel physically unwell, except when I was medication non-compliant, and even after a salutatory dose of medicine non-compliance, I only acknowledged my illness for a brief while. This perpetual inconsistency meant that, most of the time, I was profoundly, and instinctively, rejecting help. Nothing was honestly and objectively examined.

There were so many bricks in my delusional edifice, and the chapter below looks at some of them. It's a tangled mess. Where do I start? Perhaps with some emotional underpinnings. The most obvious and constant of these was my new, obsessional desire for control, which appears again and again in my story. It was at the heart of my delusional system, so it was self-evident that I was after order and structure in my life, but I didn't look for it from friends and family at the time - it was all down to me. Yes, there was a certain degree of inbuilt rigidity in my thinking, as far back as I can remember. For that reason I barely drink and I've never been drunk, but it was hardly pathological. Although it does, partially, explain my unsuccessful love life; however hard you try, you can't ever fully control how another human perceives you. It's called abuse. Ironically, nature's choice of illness for me - a total loss of control - was particularly cruel.

I'll never know why I suddenly abandoned my previous, reasonably healthy and flexible approach to life. It certainly wasn't consciously, as I'd actually been quite enjoying myself. Why was this quiet enjoyment suddenly so wrong? Yes, I made a mistake accepting the job, but it was hardly a catastrophe. In a normal, sensible world, I'd have done the job for a year or so, stayed open to other job opportunities, and enjoyed leisure activities such as creative evening classes. That's what I would have advised anyone else to do if they'd asked me for my opinion on a similar matter. Instead, I somehow slipped into a loop of endless self-punishment, to the extent that I, unconsciously, totally sabotaged that new job I was interviewed for and didn't get. It was here in this town, in this job or nothing.

The less flexible I became emotionally, partly through tiredness, the more rigid my internally generated systems became. I didn't have obsessive compulsive disorder or anorexia, but the perfectionist parallels are striking; I wasn't trying to be perfect, I was just trying to be acceptable. I worked obsessively, partly because the goblins told me to do so but partly because I was aware that my ability to function properly was slipping through my fingers. That obsessional control was mirrored in my belief system. There was no way that belief system could be dismantled until I felt more in control of my life, however hard outsiders tried to help me.

When it came to control, the most powerful and complex emotional response I felt was compulsion to believe. This compulsion made it very difficult to reason with me because it meant that I was impervious to alternative points of view. I believed, because the goblins demanded that I should believe, and they were in charge. So I did, but it wasn't straightforward. There was related anger: why should I be made to believe? There was fear: I have to believe because the goblins are all knowing and all powerful. I couldn't divorce these uncomfortable emotions from the belief structure, so tackling it was a minefield. That overarching compulsion to believe gave consistency and structure to the delusional system, and it justified and soothed the uncomfortable emotions associated with it. Which was weirdly paradoxical, as the obvious question is: 'Why are you sticking your hand in the fire and then being grateful for the ointment? Just don't put your hand in the fire in the first place ...' There's an obvious answer; I was so generally confused and upset that any structure was attractive, however injurious. If I didn't keep the faith, the whole edifice would collapse and become chaotic. It couldn't be touched.

My delusional constructs were also supported by emotionally appropriate responses - by this I don't mean that these responses were correct, I'm just saying I generally had a plausibly correct emotion for goblin instructions. If a goblin was threatening, I felt threatened. I certainly didn't think, 'Oh silly old goblins, they're off again.' Things would have been a lot easier if I had, but it literally never occurred to me to be so disrespectful.

'Disrespectful', what a word, but it was true. The goblin kingdom relied on this 'touch me not' attitude, so typical of my own behaviour in times of stress. The goblins certainly didn't encourage me to enquire too deeply, it was another of the things I was 'not allowed' to do.

In other words it was another unconsciously, self-imposed restriction to keep my delusional system viable. It was, however, a little more nuanced than a straight prohibition; it also felt almost insolent, so back to disrespectful. It's not polite to minutely examine, uninvited, other people's (or goblins') motives and reasoning. As far as I was concerned, the goblins were a secretive supernatural lot and had an entire intellectual existence I was not aware of.

As supernatural beings, any goblin theory could be, at least potentially, correct. Therefore any outsiders approaching the problem logically were at a disadvantage before they'd even begun. Goblin otherworldliness was very handy when it came to dismissing inconsistencies pointed out to me by Sean and other mental health workers, and also the inconsistencies that I came across myself. People would tell me that the goblins were in no way believable and I would think they must be, otherwise why would I believe in them? Why would I want to make them up? Who would? They were horrible. This left only the illness hypothesis, which I found suspicious, so there were, as far as I was concerned, no good reasons to realistically undermine my ideas. You couldn't ask me to analyse why the CIA might be watching me ... possible, but unlikely ... or why my neighbour wanted to kill me ... possible, and more likely, especially during the abortive plaster-removing sessions in the hall. At least neighbours and the CIA existed; there was something to hold onto. Goblins were more elusive than mercury.

There were also more practical considerations to slide around - the essence of goblins,

I guess. How do goblins really live? How did they come about in the first place, long before their involvement with me? What do they eat? How do they reproduce? Do they sleep? Are there infant goblins? Do old goblins die, or do they indeed get 'old' at all? Do they feel pain? After all, you wouldn't ask Tinkerbell if she had repetitive stress injury in her wand arm. Anything and everything. Again, it was a case of don't know, don't ask.

I did, however, know that my usual watchful goblin chaperones - or goblin prison guards, depending on my frame of mind - were only a few of the many; the many who were extremely busy on other, unspecified matters. I lived with the stress of being constantly watched by these hostile entities and my feelings were very similar to those described by victims of stalking. These included fear, suspiciousness, poor concentration, disbelief that I was in this victim situation (though sadly little disbelief as to reality of goblins), self-blame, guilt, shame, isolation and helplessness. All very reasonable responses, until you take into account that I was both stalker and victim. I was stalking myself.

This unconscious manipulation of self is normal; we all comfort ourselves with day to day fibs as it helps us manage a periodically unpleasant and unjust world. However, in psychosis it is developed to an extreme degree. For example, goblin talk sounds suspiciously akin to the way people in cults are manipulated. I find this interesting; my conscious personality would have no idea how to become a cult leader, though I guess I could come up with a few ideas on paper. Practically speaking, I'm low on charisma, my ability to manipulate people isn't great, I've zero enthusiasm for communal life and, to be honest, it all sounds too stressful anyway - quite apart from any moral considerations. However, some part of me, somewhere, would strongly disagree with this self-assessment. It knows exactly how to create a cult leader, both in theory and in practice - well, as long as it's a goblin. Unlocking one's inner potential isn't always a good thing.

Goblins would say, in so many words, that the world outside of their control was frightening and dangerous; that they were my only true friends; that I was totally dependent on them; and all the rest. That said, I wasn't always totally convinced by the 'only true friends' bit of this rhetoric. I might have seen myself as deserving of all this unpleasantness, but I was generally aware that the goblins weren't great at the friendship bit. I had real friends and they certainly didn't behave like this and, although isolation is a classic causal factor in the development of psychosis, it wasn't forced upon me by the outside world. I was not socially excluded by family, friends or colleagues. Nobody bullied me or set out to hurt me, or indeed made me feel inferior in any way. I'd never been in an abusive relationship, as I'm more than capable of walking away from that kind of trouble. So, when I told people that goblins were my only friends, it was less that I really had faith in goblins and more that I was rejecting those around me, telling them that they couldn't help me.

Victimhood, as a concept, had not previously been an acknowledged part of my adult composition and that's why it took a long time for me to realise that I was recreating myself as a victim. I unconsciously set out to destroy the good hand I'd been blessed with in life. After all, I wasn't drinking, or hurting myself, or gambling, or behaving impulsively (apart from the toxic issue of medication compliance). I couldn't be criticised for such obvious concrete things. I was, of course, more than capable of derogatory self-talk, a degree of perfectionism, plenty of self-pity and all the rest. Reinventing myself as a victim was the ultimate way out of this mess. I couldn't achieve ... whatever ... lots ... because I was a victim. I wasn't responsible for other people and their feelings ... because I was a victim. I farmed out and disowned my failures. There was no way I was consciously going to abandon this comforting, but dangerous, narrative. This was presumably one of my chief emotional investments in my delusional structure. It was a form of emotional money laundering.

These were dangerous beliefs, because instead of seeing myself as ill - and therefore fixable - I saw myself as a victim of goblins and fixing me was out of my hands. Self-governance was not my problem. So, what was the point of medication and other forms of therapy intended to help me? This is very sad, and deeply frustrating, because accepting I was the victim of an illness would have been the most sensible, and achievable, route out of the awful goblin world.

It was a disempowering narrative, a classic conspiracy theory, and because the goblins were always with me it was constantly reinforced. It persistently fed the flames of my paranoia about external reality, a paranoia I was, however erroneously, using as a malignant survival mechanism in an overwhelming world. I was a very frightened person, trapped between the imaginary, horrible goblins on one side and the real, horrible world on the other. Frightened people are very difficult to reason with. I was enthralled by fear to the extent that even benign, safe places were compromised; I was always looking out for trouble. At least goblins were generally consistent, and however unpleasant their modus operandi, they offered a simple, childlike world view. This was unsurprising, as my mental capacity to deal with broader issues was strictly limited at the time. I wasn't able to comprehend, cope with, or indeed analyse anything other than the very uncomplicated.

I think the most annoying thing anyone ever said to me on the subject (by the private psychologist, Dr A; he really knew how to get under my skin), was that, 'I believed in goblins because it made me feel special.' NO! NO! NO! In an ideal world, I'd have lent him the goblins for a few days to see how he liked it. Though I can see his logic. After all, I invented them. Believing in goblins was definitely an unusual approach to life and certainly set me apart, thereby making me feel special. Although if I'd treasured this unusualness it really would have been a good idea to choose a delusional system that the rest of the world didn't find so amusing.

I could also argue that my goblin creation - my new special friends - expressed my loneliness and relative isolation when it comes to intimate relationships. Perhaps I needed goblins as companions and guardians during a time of anxiety and uncertainty. (Just for the record, definitely not lovers; my goblins were one of the least sexy humanoid figures that anyone could come up with.) Much as I complain, I have to admit that goblins were a morbidly amplified version of my own personality, though hardly the best bits. Hence, they offered a certain degree of familiarity; they were basically my tribe. That's how they were so able to manage and manipulate me; they asked me to do things I could uncomfortably fit into my world view and definitely not things I could never imagine doing at all. Back to sex again, although sexual perversions were never mentioned by the goblins, thankfully.

Stockholm Syndrome also comes to mind when looking at my emotional investment in goblins. I was certainly hostile to well-meaning outsiders trying to help me and I was, in a weird way, a sort of parent to the goblins. For all the goblin talk of omniscience and omnipotence, they were even more useless than boastful children when it came to coping with the real world, i.e. the world outside me. I was their protector, and I was the one facilitating communication; a sort of Harry Corbett to a bunch of delinquent goblin puppets. So goblins needed protecting, this protected the delusional structure and, in a very poisonous way, protected me from the nasty real world.

There are two further considerations: pride and power. When

looking at subconscious motivations, I also have to ask whether I clung onto goblin beliefs for so long to protect myself from loss of face? This is a tricky one, because if I had admitted I was wrong about goblins, I would have looked like a fool. Yet by continuing to believe in goblins, I looked like a fool anyway. When I told people I was optionless, this might have been an example. Exit routes out of a delusional world are torturous and obscure.

Then, there's power. For all my complaints about feeling powerless and victimised, did the goblins make me feel powerful in an overwhelming world? After all, through goblins I could control conversations, I could set the rules: my private goblin rules that I was happy to express but no one else was privileged to really understand. Perhaps that's why the enforced hospital admissions were so profoundly upsetting. With goblins I thought that I held all the cards, and suddenly, I was thwarted. It wasn't something I was aware of consciously ... but unconsciously? Who's to say.

Certainly, CBT techniques and other approaches didn't really work for me, as I was never fully prepared to wholly accept examination and moderation of my internal thought processes. If the external logic is not matched by an internal response from the patient, there's basically not much point. The idea of a therapeutic partnership couldn't have been further from goblin totalitarian ideology and, while I did have a therapeutic relationship with Sean, I always held a certain amount of myself back. I wasn't aware I was doing this but, for a long time, my innermost core was mostly impregnable. It was my little, secret, place of power. That figures, considering the way my illness manifested itself through pathological control.

How much I shared later with family and friends is hazy, but of course people outside mental services tried to help me. However, nobody close to me, those people I loved and trusted, could shake my delusional construct. They would ask me sensible questions like:

'If you didn't believe in goblins before, how come you believe in them now?'

To which the obvious answer was, 'Well, that was because they did exist; it was something I just wasn't aware of previously.'

Game, set and match to me. I was very good at cul de sac responses when it came to awkward questions.

The furious poet, no longer so furious, was very kind and we went for long walks and watched films. The balance of power had changed here, as I was far less the self-sufficient, proud person I'd been and he was also curious about my psychotic world. He was obviously trying to help me but I, typically, seem to have rejected this help. In November 2001 he was evicted from his flat. According to my medical notes, it was, apparently, the fault of the goblins as they were, 'exacting revenge for him saying the goblins were lying.' Really? It wasn't as though my goblin explanation was filling a void - he'd told me why he was being evicted and it was entirely plausible (he'd had an argument with the landlord). So, yet again, I pushed someone else's truth to one side to fit my own, questionable, narrative.

Sadly, I had very little understanding or even empathy when it came to interacting with other people at this time and rarely acknowledged their feelings, quite apart from their more helpfully conventional beliefs. To put it bluntly, I had to keep people away from the heart of the delusional system if I wanted to keep it intact. Not that I realised this at the time; it's only looking back I can now understand why I wouldn't let people help me. It was literally too dangerous - at least within my framework. Therefore, subconsciously, how much did I really want to be helped? Everything was too scary.

My interpretation of the furious (or by now, more friendly) poet's accommodation woes was typical of my reasoning when more unwell. I would project my goblin world onto other people; they were controlled by goblins, or at least affected by goblins, but they just didn't know it. If you really want to annoy people try this experiment; it's very rewarding. I, however, was never quite sure what I'd done wrong. Why were people so cross with me?

Now, I realise that I was effectively telling them that any help they were offering me was not only ineffectual but totally useless, and that they didn't know their own minds, or rather thought they did, but didn't. And that I, the oh, so successful (hmm ...) patient, family member or friend, depending on who I was talking to, knew far more about the world than they did. When you're talking to a psychiatrist, for example, who has trained for years and has a higher IQ than you, this comes across as not only deeply deluded but extremely arrogant as well. I apologise; as ever this was more about me than whoever was at the receiving end of this theory. That said, it did conveniently deflect awkward questions about goblins.

Certainly, getting me to take responsibility for the evil goblin thoughts was impossible.

I 'didn't have' these awful thoughts and I knew they were wrong, therefore it was the goblins' bright ideas, not mine. My argument here was that I hadn't had these thoughts prior to the goblins, so they must be generated by goblins (definite proof, by the way, that goblins really existed). The counter argument was that I did have the thoughts before, I just wasn't aware of them.

Just imagine how that counter argument feels when you're on the receiving end. It's incredibly annoying and distressing. After all, I'd been living in the world, reasonably successfully for thirty years, so, of course I knew what thoughts I did, or did not have. What right did other people to tell me that I didn't? As far as I was concerned, my life with the goblins was horrible, without being told I was responsible for their more dangerously antisocial views as well. Why was I being asked to take on someone else's - i.e. the goblins' - unhealthy and unpleasant belief structure? Yet, when I told helpful outsiders that they, themselves, were influenced by goblins, but were unaware of this interesting fact, I was using exactly the same argument, with no justification at all. No wonder they were fed up; they weren't seeking help from me ... In my defence, my self-esteem, what was left of it, demanded that these evil thoughts were not mine, so I was using the delusional system as a protection of last resort. 'Everything's a truly horrible mess,' I thought, 'but at least those evil thoughts have nothing to do with me.'

It also rarely occurred to me that there was no way anyone outside me could know what was going on in the goblin world, unless I told them everything from A to Z, and not just by giving them a random selection of bits and pieces and expecting them to get on with it. (This seems to have been an inbuilt failing, as my father says that, as a small child, I expected him to fit jigsaw pieces together in the order I presented them to him.) Therefore, risk assessing me was challenging. As far as I was concerned, I'd already told mental health services everything about the goblins' more lurid ambitions, hadn't I? If there was anything new I'd tell them. OK ... Except how was the unfortunate interviewer supposed to know that? How were they supposed to know I was being truthful? How could they know, that while I might not have acted on threats from last week, I might be making concrete plans for murdering people the next? How could they possibly work out how the goblins were feeling? Or, by implication, how homicidal I was feeling. Or how arsonical and so forth. This was a fundamental problem. I could hardly undermine my delusional structure, if I couldn't even truly grasp that it was unique to me - and impossible for others to access without asking me - and, even worse, that there was even a delusional structure to undermine. My failure to understand this made me incredibly difficult to treat, as most of the time I had no idea why people were asking me various questions and why they were making certain high-handed, as I saw it, decisions about my care.

For psychiatrists, in particular, this was a worry. They had to work out how dangerous I was. 'Dangerous? I'm not dangerous, that's the goblins, not me,' was my very unhelpful default position. What did I expect psychiatrists to do? Interview the goblins without me?

I wonder ... After all, the psychiatrists would be considered partly accountable if I'd achieved some of my bloodier desires.

Not that I understood this at all at the time, as it was many, many years before I truly understood that psychiatrists were real people, with feelings and anxieties of their own, and even a life beyond their consulting rooms. Of course, I knew all this in theory but, practically speaking, childish me viewed them (whether male or female) as sort of demonic headmasters who had to be resisted. After all, they fed me nasty medicines and sometimes, inexplicably and unfairly, interfered in my life. That said, I'm sure some psychiatrists (and other mental health workers) would have loved to have banished me to a corner of the room until I'd written, at least a thousand times: 'I must take antipsychotic medication.' Or, 'If I do not take antipsychotic medication, I will become even more psychotic. Discuss.' I wouldn't blame them. I only saw Sean once, years ago, after leaving the northern town, and I remember apologising for my medication avoidance. 'It must have driven you mad,' I said. 'You could say that,' he replied, somewhat diplomatically.

I also never understood why psychiatrists and other mental health professionals were perpetually asking me if I understood the consequences of command hallucinations. It was intensely frustrating and annoying. I was perfectly clear, I thought, when I said other people would be disastrously hurt or, at worst, die. I knew I'd end up in a secure hospital, so why keep asking me? Yet, I saw no contradiction whatsoever, when I sometimes, almost simultaneously, announced that whatever I did the goblins would look after me. This was because I was doing their bidding; or I would become a goblin myself; or my victims would become goblins and as a result 'wouldn't mind' being dead. Did I really think that becoming a goblin was the pinnacle of anyone's desire, including my own? I don't know, but it was yet another convenient and muddled dead end to the conversation.

Unfortunately, this meant that psychiatric appointments became very repetitive, as we went over and over the same distressing and depressing assessment and analysis of my 'bad' thoughts. Consequently, my delusional structure was always being strengthened and revalidated. Would the thoughts have been more fleeting otherwise? Would I have been less risky? Would I have felt less dangerous and unhappy and hence the thoughts would have been less violent? I don't know the answer to any of these questions and if I don't know myself, even now, it must have been virtually impossible for outsiders. I was usually treated considerately and sometimes compassionately as well - I can see that from the medical notes - but, unfortunately, I became like Pavlov's dog. I only had to catch sight of a psychiatrist and I was off again about the bad intentions of the goblins. That was all that psychiatrists were interested in, weren't they? The poor psychiatrists would then note that I only would talk about goblins. We were, possibly, at cross-purposes here.

Psychiatric interviews were always an ordeal, particularly when my belief system was challenged. I felt persecuted by outsiders, especially when they were telling me not to believe in goblins and were pointing out all sorts of inconsistencies, however correctly. I felt that I was always having to defend goblins from the sceptical and make excuses for their unreliable nature, while, at the same time, defending my own 'unreasonable' views. Initially, the goblins' commands were relatively innocuous; they didn't, for example, ask me to burn down the museum or kill Sean. That all came later. In fact the goblins themselves never really evolved at all; they remained primitive or perhaps basic. My ideas about their potential for evil flourished, though. To what extent did I 'upgrade' their evil activities as a defensive response to all those people who were attacking my delusional structure, and even as a defensive response to myself? I genuinely tried not to believe in goblins. Later on, I started linking goblins with the Devil. How much was this an attempt by me to convince outsiders, and myself, that these creatures were as truly evil as I believed and stated aloud?

Then there was the muddled business of visual and auditory hallucinations, which I've tried to explain in chapter six. These were supported by all sorts of perceptual inconsistencies.

For example, it's been suggested, entirely plausibly, that in schizophrenia recognition and identification of the always active, inner voice fails, but I found it impossible to identify quite how the failure worked. It wasn't as though my non-goblin inner voice ceased. It was still able to deal with everyday life, from the mundane, 'I think I'll buy some tomatoes,' to the deeper, 'I wonder what so and so meant when they said that?' Although it's possible, looking back, that there was less non-goblin inner speech; not so much in amount but more in content, as I focussed obsessively on goblins and my present predicament. So while I must have incorrectly reassigned some of my inner voice activity to the goblins, it didn't feel as though I had, and it was a difficult concept for me to accept. Which bits had I unconsciously reassigned? How was it sorted out in my brain?

Once those auditory neural pathways were set up, things became even more complicated. Nothing, now, was unreasonable. I could, and still can, manufacture goblin instructions out of ambient non-specific noise, patterns of silence, rustling leaves blown across a pavement, anything really. It's well known that the brain can be tricked into hearing almost anything in white noise, but it didn't happen so specifically to me (i.e. reliably productive of goblin voices) before I was ill. These internal goblin voices, and as a result internal instructions, I would unconsciously identify as externally generated. After all, the triggering leaf sounds, or whatever, came from outside, didn't they? Therefore, it made perfect sense to me that the information, or instructions embodied within them, were equally external.

This was the same with visual hallucinations. It was easy for me to keep the goblins visible while I looked at them; there was no conscious work involved. So, it made it difficult for me to understand these visions as being the product of my mind's eye. If I want to, my mind's eye can populate anywhere with anything. That's a normal brain function. I can imagine a large, lively spider scuttling across the floor, and while I know that's a perfectly possible sight, I know it's not really there, so I won't squeak and lift up my feet.

More pertinently, I can also select something less likely. Just for fun, I've 'put' a small zebra in front of my kitchen door as I'm writing this paragraph. I can dress it up with a few activities to make it more real - it's scuffing its hooves on the mat and whinnying. So, now there's imaginary noise too but, in spite of this, I'm one hundred percent clear that it's a totally imaginary visitor, purely created by me, and that's not only because it's largely transparent and I have to work hard to keep it there for any length of time. I know it's not there because why would there be a zebra in my living room? It's ridiculous. I don't even own a goldfish.

But it *was* possible for my brain to put even more ridiculous goblins all over the place, without any apparent input from me at all. That's partly why I was so convinced they were real. At no point, did I ever consciously say, 'I know, I think my life would be greatly improved by some nasty, ugly, little, green men things.' It was presumably my unconscious brain that thought this was a good idea.

That said, although the 'sighting' of goblins came easily, there were still big issues with my 'reality' theory, which I carefully skated around. My mind's eye, or unconscious mind wasn't really up to creating proper, solid 3D. This incongruity was supported by my fearful refusal to physically touch the goblins. However, if I had and found them to be no more than gauzy visions, I would have argued that this was because they were semi-supernatural - friends of ghosts and other such transparent things.

There was also a strong degree of expectation. Once they were an established part of my world view, I saw goblins when I expected to see them - and struggled far more to 'create' them in less typical places; the hospital comes to mind here. Some people have their TV in the corner of the room; I had random goblins. I had categorised them as not liking warm, brightly lit, modern places, so supermarkets, for example, were entirely goblin-free.

While the goblins insisted I ate only cold food (cold damp food, cold damp house, it sort of fits together) my actual shopping basket was never scrutinised. Not that it really mattered. Obedient me just bought things on the 'approved' shopping list anyway.

Many sightings were entirely devoid of meaningful content, and were probably no more than a habit, a sort of accidental brain training. I would then give these sightings an unwarranted significance; these goblins weren't just empty shadows, they were actually busy 'watching', a good catch all explanation for what was essentially 'just hanging about purpose unspecified', in the kind of places I'd expect to see them.

I also never examined, or even considered, how many goblins they were in total (apart from the initial and relatively brief ascendency of the 'council of twelve.') Did I see the same goblins over and over again, or were they different goblins every time? Who knows, it was another conveniently vague area. It was incredibly difficult for an outsider, quite apart from me, to take apart this nebulous tangle of goblins who could, potentially, be anywhere, and in any number.

As with auditory hallucinations, when I was (or am) unwell, I obsessively looked for visual patterns with encoded information: such as raindrops against a window, or the criss-crossing dark and light shadows of a conifer hedge. This didn't happen before my illness. However, I have never discovered any meaning in these patterns at all. This should ring warning bells; perhaps there aren't any patterns to be decoded but, no ... the information is there somewhere. I'm just too thick to uncover it properly. I'm still searching for reassuring order and meaning, and using it to overlay puzzling or alarming reality.

Finally, what were the goblins up to when I couldn't see or hear them? I offered no challengeable theories to either myself or outsiders, other than a vague, 'they were snaring the unwary with a view to exploiting them.' This lack of clarity also gave me a convenient explanation for my own windows of sanity. It meant I could carry out a particular forbidden act (forbidden by the goblins, not by me, obviously) because 'the goblins weren't looking'. They were somehow busy elsewhere and, after all, they had other things to do than worry about me. Which was sort of true, as I wasn't summoning them up to interfere.

As a result of all this auditory and visual vagueness, I've subsequently looked into pseudo- hallucinations and, as ever, found a number of not entirely consistent definitions. However, apart from the very important fact that I don't think I have true auditory or visual hallucinations, in other ways I do seem to have fitted some of the criteria for true hallucinations. I did not perceive goblin instructions and intrusions subjectively; they were usually objective experiences. I did not understand that the goblins were perceptually inconsistent. I did have some insight, but it tended to be overridden by my more attention demanding abnormal thought processes and was, therefore, fluctuating. The hallucinations were internally consistent in that they fitted in with my delusional structure. Overall, goblin hallucinations or pseudo-hallucinations were not substantively different in content and meaning from the true externally heard or sighted hallucinations. Neither were they transitory. I was stuck with them for years.

So all these ins and outs made attempts to undermine the goblin world, or rather my delusional world, by outsiders, or even me, very difficult. I would sometimes accept a degree of moderation when I was talking to someone but, as soon as their back was turned, the compulsion to believe at all costs had the upper hand. There are a lot of references in the notes to my goblin views being shakeable, but sadly this 'shakeability' was transitory and disappeared when the voice of reason - Sean, or whoever - left me to my own devices. This perpetual inconsistency must have made me very awkward to treat and, as a result, I frequently felt as though I was caught in a low level therapeutic war. People interviewing me probably felt the same way. Sadly, the goblins really did have an answer for everything.

CHAPTER 14 LAST SEEN

2nd November 2000, Sean, telephone call:

> *Jane was initially quite negative and stated if the wicked thoughts left her, what would be left of her as she feels she is nothing without them.*

What do you do if someone steals your identity? You speak to the police, you speak to various official bodies attempting to discover the extent of the fraud, and attempt to contain it, and all the other sensible things to do. Now, imagine your identity has been hijacked by some entities that nobody else believes in. What do you do? Ring the fairyland support line? It's a big problem. These entities won't empty your bank account but they'll empty your life, and all you'll end up with is a blister pack of pills. Just look at the pills; they're no more than tiny white disks. The goblins are all knowing, all controlling beings and they're hardly going to be ameliorated by something so insignificant.

Schizophrenia generally causes a profound disturbance in the patient's comprehension of self. Before I was ill, I had no issues at all with knowing who I was both physically and mentally. I realise that this is an illusion; the self varies from moment to moment depending on what's happening both internally and externally, and the stable sense of self I enjoyed was a generalisation. I was physically very well and followed basically sensible rules about diet and exercise to support this. My appearance caused me no more than the usual anxieties. How I dressed and presented myself didn't alter much over the years. There were no dramatic transformations and the word reinvention wasn't in my vocabulary. My external shell was essentially nondescript.

Mentally, I had fairly consistent views and opinions about myself and who I was, and these fundamental views and opinions didn't change much, whoever I was with and whatever the situations I found myself in. For example, I always voted for the same political party as, while I sometimes disagreed strongly with particular details of their policies, I was broadly in agreement with their principles.

My interests and friendships were generally stable. I didn't make friends easily and I've never been popular, but there are enough people in the world who share my interests and/or values, so I've never been totally isolated. I wasn't bullied at school but there wasn't a lot of bullying at my school anyway. I still see a school friend and she told me, recently, that girls would occasionally ask her why I did this, that, or another, and my friend would respond: 'What's it to you, she's not doing any harm?' In return, I would shove her if she fell asleep in A Level English; her life was much more interesting and therefore exhausting than mine. She's still a good friend.

So, my identity and self-image were, as far as I understood it, secure. If you had told me what was going to happen, I'd have said: 'You what? Me?' and felt distinctly misunderstood, unfairly assessed and very puzzled. As far as I was concerned, I had a capable but not outstanding brain (my university was mid-league Russell Group) that usually delivered what I asked of it, provided I wasn't too ambitious. This academically competent background was matched by a reasonably competent, adult lifestyle. Things had been a little difficult in my late teens but that had been processed and dealt with a long time ago, although there were a few unhappy echoes when I was reviewing my CV.

I took this tidy life for granted. I had no need of counselling, helplines or any extra support.
To be honest, I worked quite hard to keep worries under control and, like most of us, had ups and downs but, on the whole, I was happy. I didn't always like parts of my character, but who does? My only major regret was inability to maintain intimate

relationships; my love life had been a bit of a disaster, but it was a case of so be it. There was no point dwelling on things.

This was the situation before I was ill. Reasonable equilibrium. That was why, when things started to fall apart, I was so clueless. I had no previous history of delusions or perceptual abnormalities at all, unlike many schizophrenics who can recall such episodes, sometimes as far back as their childhood. As an enthusiastic reader, particularly of psychological fiction, I was interested in mental illness in general - but in an abstract, rather than a personal way. Unfortunately, the famous 1948 lunatic asylum film, *The Snakepit,* had totally terrified teenage me (more than any horror novel), and I'd also owned a copy of Mary Jane Ward's original book, which I'd found on a market stall. I'm sure neither helped me in my subsequent encounters with mental health services ... but, overall, the whole mental illness issue wasn't on my personal radar. It was this lack of awareness that helps explain why I fell straight into the 'heffalump' trap. I really didn't see it coming.

Looking back, however, there was one aspect of distinct disequilibrium and this did cause me some underlying concern, but no more than that. I was aware that my emotional side was generally separate from my intellectual side and I was used to jettisoning troublesome emotions, rather than working through them. I don't think it's an unusual state of affairs; it was how I'd been brought up and this must apply to a lot of people. How many times do grown-ups tell children to not be ruled by their feelings? A child has to learn to do that to survive. As this approach worked for the first thirty years of my life, I accepted that while it wasn't ideal, this was how I ran things. I couldn't imagine life with the intellectual and emotional sides of my personality in a happy symbiotic relationship, and I certainly never dreamt that this division would eventually upset the boat altogether.

Intellectual me had all sorts of positive characteristics: it achieved, it interacted positively with the outside world - both people and events, it was intelligent, it used its time reasonably well, it took sensible risks and, when in charge, my life usually went quite well. But it had a clear downside; it was very judgemental of me and others, and especially the failings of emotional me.

Emotional me had plenty of positive characteristics, but intellectual me was very dismissive of these and preferred to concentrate on the negatives. These negatives included anxiety, a tendency to cry, shyness, anger, stubbornness, neediness, hopelessness, jealousy, moodiness and general contrariness - all common negatives of the human condition, but with a strong bias towards anxiety and introversion. Finally, there was childishness. Childish, emotional me was happier in a more structured paternalistic environment. She was small and unsophisticated so, when it came to goblins, did she just get it wrong? Was it that I was always going to run into trouble when I had too much autonomy? Emotional, childish me had ambushed the competent, intellectual me in the past, but that had been tolerable, as intellectual me had previously regrouped and taken back control. Crisis averted.

Not this time. Perhaps, if I'd walked away from the town and the job at the beginning, I might have spent a definable period of time possibly depressed and then regrouped and continued. Maybe, maybe not. Perhaps the first domino in the line had already fallen. Either way, I'd been treating my emotions as an enemy that needed to be suppressed and I didn't have enough mental resources to keep it up. My old, trusted friend, intellectual me, futilely battled for supremacy; its previously positive values, of drive and discipline, were increasingly subverted and morbidly overvalued. It was a vicious circle. The repeated failure drove my negative emotions and my negative emotions drove my failure.

As these negative emotions became too strong to be easily dismissed, I guess, unconsciously, I had to work out a new role for them. This was the foundation stone of my psychosis.

Firstly, 'The Rules', these were punitive; I was punishing myself for uncontrolled negative emotions. Then came the goblins, who were also punitive but altogether weirder. So, now there were three: intellectual me, emotional me, and goblins - erm ... naturally.

Here's Sean, again, 1st February 2002, just before I left the northern town and after two years of psychiatric treatment. He was completing his final handover to other members of the local mental health service:

> *Cognitively. Jane can work through/discuss her thoughts quite rationally. States at times she has an emotional and intellectual side to herself and can differentiate between 'real and imagined', but emotionally feels their presence most of the time. No insight.*

That's such a frustrating paragraph to read. I was nearly there, within touching distance of sanity, but couldn't quite bring goblins into a place where they could be meaningfully examined. When I first read this paragraph, I was surprised that I was able to differentiate between real and not real as it's not what I remembered at all. Then I read it again, more carefully, and realised it actually says that **I said** I could ... not that I actually could. Even so, the 'at times' is correct, as when speaking to someone I trusted I could be less defensive and more open to outside suggestions. However, you really can't get past the concluding 'no insight' comment. It's pretty damning.

My introverted, self-reliant lifestyle was no help, whatsoever. If you're used to relying on yourself for support and not usually discussing problems with others, learning how to manage external help is difficult. My lack of very close relationships meant that the ideas that fed into the delusional structure went unchallenged and, as a result, flourished during that baffling and disquieting autumn of 1999. It was my big secret.

During this time, the goblins spread like cancer. They wormed their way, insidiously, throughout my brain, becoming embedded in memory, emotion, visual, and information systems. I had no comprehension of the extent to which I was being compromised. By the time I was in contact with mental health services, the damage was already well underway, and the goblins were imprinted on my body, my mind and my soul. My taken for granted self, had disastrously disintegrated. As a result, I believed that these new, and surprising, goblin visitors were extremely aggressive external invaders and certainly not generated by me.

This lack of awareness meant that my own perception of my basic self, at least at that point, was that it was mostly unchanged. I was still Jane, if a rather knocked about and increasingly diminished version, and what was left of me was, mostly, functioning the way it had been for thirty years. After all, the less elusive definitions of who exactly I was remained exactly the same: which toothpaste flavour I preferred or my favourite colour - the green I'd chosen for my front room. There was no way I'd have chosen bubble-gum pink. If I'd liked pink more, would I have ended up with fairies, or rogue Barbies, rather than goblins? Discuss. Less minutely particular, I still loved my family and appreciated my friends. I recognised that there were problems in my brain - I couldn't sleep or concentrate - but saw these as a reaction to external pressures, rather than there being something wrong in the way my brain was functioning.

However, there was absolutely no way that I could be unaware that other people believed my new identity to be totally wrong. Being told that yourself, your identity, was not how you, as its owner perceived it, was profoundly upsetting and mystifying. Had I unknowingly lapsed into some form of error mode? Had I gone mutant? If I could have agreed with outsiders looking in, I would have done so. I'm not that intransigent. Instead, it felt as though they were trying to spiritually disembowel me. If I was wrong, and the goblins were wrong, what, precisely, remained?

My response was usually defensive: my lack of compliance with medication is a good example. If you lose the ability to correctly assess yourself from the outside, how do you know you're ill? If I had been more trusting and less paranoid, I would have been easier to treat, but psychosis is a profoundly isolating disease. Normal rules don't apply, and only you, the patient, have an idea of what the new internal rules are and how liable they were to change arbitrarily. I was incapable of engaging successfully with the outside world, because I'd been tricked by my brain. My internal world was shaping my external world, to the extent it was eliminating external realities and replacing them with chimaeras. We all do this, we're hardly dispassionate observers of the external scene, but most of us, and me prior to my illness, manage to observe and react with the outside world in a manner that is broadly understood by those around us. It also enables us to fit into our chosen society and manage life successfully; hold down a job, have a family and all the rest.

Believing in and following the instructions of goblins alienated me from this entire process of pleasant self-validation. Nobody, but me, believed in goblins even after undergoing the benefits of my special knowledge and nobody, but me, had to follow the bizarre goblin rules, which were, of course, totally mysterious to outsiders, both in form and content. I was in a religion of one that I didn't remember choosing at all, and it was a very lonely place.

I was cut off from the hobbies and interests that had enriched my life and my vocationally satisfying job, which I'd worked so hard to achieve, just slipped away. Away from work, I was effectively isolated from my family and friends, because I had a new, and to them, inexplicable agenda. Yes, I could talk to them and socialise on a superficial level, but my inner preoccupations were rarely presented for inspection and, more tellingly, never moderated. I was more and more severed from real life, at the very time I needed it most to balance my obsessive introspection. My much trusted and relied upon inner world had totally failed me.

It was a weird, disturbing place to find myself in. However much I supported or believed in the goblins, I couldn't ignore the fact that my life was increasingly unfamiliar and uncomfortable. Belief in goblins was hardly a wild success. My much-loved autonomy was on the one hand sacrificed to mental health services and on the other hand to goblins. The interface between the two was distinctly painful, as mental health service facts and goblin facts were not in the least compatible. I was forever desperately trying to integrate both, while trying to hang on to an increasingly diminished me. It felt like a war, where I was standing in no man's land, unsure of how I got there, and with skirmishes going on over my head that I was in no way responsible for. To outsiders it looked as though I was absorbed in an intense, internal world, but it actually felt as though I was fighting to prevent myself from being dissolved into a hostile, external world.

That's why psychosis is so dangerous. It's as though your brain, your very core, doesn't really belong to you at all, which makes it very difficult to repair. How could I fix a brain that was everyone else's property? I knew that if I felt depressed, I could accept that my low spirits were something to do with my brain chemistry, and depending on severity, a good walk, change of approach, or medication might help. Simple. But how do you know what to do when the responsibility for the 'self-function' of your busy, busy brain seems to have been stolen from you, when you weren't paying attention?

That's what it felt like - an unreasonable task. There's no doubt that mental health services worked hard to establish a trusting, working relationship with me; I have their notes as evidence. But at the same time I had the ever-present goblins telling me to trust them, that they were my only friends, and even that they 'owned' me. Their constant presence gave them access to me and my thought processes whenever they wanted, twenty four hours a day. No wonder I was influenced by them, and my internal world trumped the external world. I'd have to have been a far braver, more robust character to resist.

It felt awful. I was watching my life disintegrate and I couldn't fix it. I believed that I myself wanted to re-engage with my life, but was this really true? If it was, why had I put the goblins in charge? I was attacking my sense of self through them, without even realising it. As a result, especially near the beginning, I was angry, resentful and bewildered. I didn't remember signing up for this at all. I seemed to be trapped in a never-ending horror movie. Those late night films, the kind of fantasies we watch in a fairly detached way, were suddenly, dreadfully true.

The goblins had shut down the escape routes and I felt totally optionless. Optionless ... this word appears again and again, in my notes. Why was I shutting down myself? Why was I walking away and abandoning me? In psychosis, this isn't a metaphorical state of affairs, it's literal. That's what you're doing. It's gradual internal suicide. I was attempting to murder my self and I didn't understand this in the slightest, because the goblins were the aggressors, not me.

As I offered myself no escape routes, of course my situation was increasingly desperate. As time went on I felt more and more hopeless and empty. My coherent, centred self - the one I used to take for granted - was now weak and starved. The parasitical goblins had sucked it dry, taking strength from my energy. In other words, instead of taking strength from the external world, I was feeding solely on my internal world. It was a form of cannibalism. With this enfeebled self, I knew I could never win back the control I had so prized. I didn't have the weapons. I knew that, fundamentally, I would never be a good enough goblin 'slave'. However many babies I killed, it would never be enough. If I burnt down the museum then the goblins would be lining up the next target for my arson. If I sold my house and gave away my money, they'd be eyeing up the clothes on my back. The only way out of this mess was suicide, and I wasn't even brave enough for that.

Eventually, I believed that my identity was totally shattered. For a while, I felt totally subsumed. I didn't know myself at all. All my memories, my life experiences, my personality, my achievements were meaningless. It was as though 'I' had never actually existed. I was so out of touch with reality, that I believed that goblin talk and actions were not about me at all. I was just an unwilling conduit. I didn't realise that they clearly indicated how I myself was feeling. I was letting the goblins do the talking ... Even my physical body image was changed; if I held out my arms I didn't see human arms, I saw greenish brown, twiggy goblin arms. This was the future. Me, myself, was gone, destroyed. I didn't exist anymore.

Only I do exist, and I always did. I'd been trapped in a maelstrom of confused thoughts and perceptions. I'd lost sight of the boundaries between real and imaginary, between where I myself started and where I myself finished. I was totally alienated from everything. I do sometimes still visit this place but never voluntarily. It's not fun. I don't get blinding flashes of altered consciousness, where I'm in harmony with the world and able to perceive in totality its beauty and knowledge. If I did, I'm not sure I'd have sought treatment in the first place. Altered consciousness, as far as I was concerned, was a frightening, bleak, confusing place, and extremely damaging to everyday life. Psychosis and creativity may well be linked for some people, but they're usually bipolar. Anything starting with 'schizo' is bad news if you're hoping madness will touch you with genius.

There's still a part of me that's looking for the person I was. I imagine going back to the northern town, and visiting my old house in search of the Jane I knew; she could be there, wandering about looking for her body. If I really thought that was a possibility I'd be up there now, clutching my flashlight for the hours of darkness. But that complete person's gone irrevocably because Jane, for all her faults, never doubted her perception of herself. In fact, she never even gave the issue a second thought, having nothing but passing interests in philosophical and medical matters. She never worried that if she got too stressed (this seems to be the principal problem) everything could, all of a sudden, get very weird indeed.

Yes, I do know that the pre-illness person still lives within me, though now she's a sort of recycled version made of bits and pieces of me, picked up and jammed together, haphazardly. It was the best I could do in the circumstances and my new self usually gets on reasonably well. It has held down a job, followed interests and hobbies, has reasonable concentration, kept friends and appreciates and loves the family. It's not a spectacular life, but at least it's mine … usually.

CHAPTER 15 BABIES

If there was one thing that really bothered psychiatrists, it was my frequently expressed desire to kill babies. Fortunately for me, and especially everybody else, my sedate, drug and alcohol-free lifestyle was a protective factor. Substance abuse, in particular, is a well-known causative factor when it comes to acting on command hallucinations.

That said, what I did say was alarming, though not deliberately so. I didn't set out to shock or make these claims because I was seeking attention. I expressed them because I felt they needed to be said; goblins were evil and dangerous and this was indisputable proof. I didn't feel it would be responsible to keep quiet. However, luckily for me, I didn't go around broadcasting this theory more widely because I was selfishly and deeply ashamed that the goblins had selected me for these appalling acts.

'Babies are evil and must be eliminated,' the goblins announced, thereby leaving me with a schedule somewhat fuller than King Herod's ... Should I be flippant? What's funny about baby killing? Or threatened baby killing? Nothing. Evil is a very visceral term, it's very absolute in its condemnation, and what on earth had babies done to deserve this? Basically, I don't know ... so the best I can do is talk around the problem. Something was obviously seriously wrong somewhere; one baby would be bad enough, but all of them? Really?

The first baby 'victim' belonged to a close friend, mass infanticide came later. When it came to the baby of my friend, I assume I was jealous because I felt, correctly, that the baby would partially usurp our friendship. I'm guessing I was fearfully envisaging an emotional life without her support. Maybe this reminded me of losing the automatic protection of my parents as I grew up. Did I want the safety and security of being a baby, to be looked after myself? Or was it simply that my friendship with her had been a happy time and losing this easy relationship was another thing, amongst so many, that was slipping through my fingers.

However, those rationalisations came later. At the time, I was totally unable to identify the root of my hostility towards this particular baby and found the whole affair deeply distressing and puzzling. My inability to achieve a longer, more objective view was disastrous; there was no way I could work through these unwanted and unfamiliar feelings. I wouldn't have been proud of them but, as humans, we have all sorts of automatic reactions that make us think: 'Oh, bloody hell, better remove that one to the back burner!'

Jealousy is hugely important to my story. It's not a pretty emotion and definitely one not to be proud of. It's not easy, however, to recall those memories of jealousy in my unremarkable, happy childhood. In fact, it's a weird quest. Why would I want to revive childhood slights? They don't bother me now, at least not consciously. I know I wasn't a warm, caring older sister; I was more like the cross-grained, big sister Katy in Susan Coolidge's classic children's novel *What Katy Did* - before she had the life-changing accident and reinvented herself as 'good.'

In spite of this, I loved and still love all my siblings, and I can't imagine life without them. All our family relationships are essentially harmonious, we're that kind of family. Having a childhood of ready-made playmates, even though some of them were rather small, was fantastic and I remember so much fun, noise and happiness. It was our own private world. How lucky we were. My school friends' homes felt very quiet and empty; I'd be tiptoeing about, self-conscious and suddenly, uncomfortably aware of grown up lives.

However, the more I try, the more I remember. I was definitely a jealous child, hopefully not pathologically so, but that possibility can't be ruled out. As the oldest child in my family, I learnt from an early age that there was always someone younger and cuter than me. I would also have to earn praise for good schoolwork, or whatever, whereas, as I saw it, a younger sibling would be the centre of attention just because they were adorable. Adorable? Not as far as I was concerned, at least when I was a child. Younger siblings were also exempt from the rules we older ones had to follow; unsurprisingly, over the years, these rules were increasingly discarded by our exhausted parents.

More profoundly, I do remember being in trouble periodically for failing to reconcile my roles as both child and adult. I had a tendency to be overbearing and this was discouraged by my parents, who scolded me for taking on an adult role to which I was not entitled. However, at the same time I was expected to keep an eye on younger siblings, and make sure the little darlings didn't stick their fingers in bicycle spokes or consume poisonous odds and ends in the garden. If I neglected to do so I wasn't being adult enough although, for the record, under my somewhat casual care nobody came to much harm, possibly because taking babies and toddlers into account became second nature. I was not emotionally sophisticated, so I struggled with this contradiction and sometimes felt very hard done by indeed. 'It's not fair, not fair,' I'd complain bitterly, just as I did later when the goblins made my life miserable, even though I'd heard the obvious response a thousand times. 'Life's not fair,' my parents would say. They were right, it isn't and many people have far more to deal with than me, but I found this scrap of life wisdom very annoying. Why was I being asked to consider the plight of a starving, distant child? The emotional impact of my minor domestic upset was here and now, and much more overwhelming and important.

Growing up was sometimes tricky. When I was a teenager the family's focus, inevitably, was primarily centred on meeting the needs of younger children. It occasionally felt as though I was pushed out of childhood pleasures, the, 'oh you're too big, why do you want to join in with this ...?' I sometimes found this very difficult, as I took comfort from routine and remembered pleasures. There was a small part of me that would have been happy enough to be a child forever, without having to brave the frightening outside world.

My parents, however, were keen for me to develop as an adult. There was no question of that, and I agreed. Until the advent of the goblins, I was living a conventional adult life. I certainly don't consciously remember more than a passing desire to return to childhood after I left home for university 200 miles away. At university, I remember house-sharing with a girl who phoned her parents every night, but I spoke to my parents about once a month, although I did sometimes exchange letters with my mother (no emails in those days). So, achieving adulthood might have been sometimes painful but being there was fine, and I did not consciously want, or even envisage, my sudden, inglorious return to semi-childhood.

Many of the goblin commands and certainly their method of delivery, were, however, infantilising. Was I attempting to regain the safety and security of childhood? If I were, it was a very warped childhood indeed. I can see some goblin parallels in my upbringing but those juvenile woes were amplified exponentially. The goblins were never good parents to me. Had they been helpful, or at the very least comforting, I doubt I'd have ever come into contact with mental health services. They were more 'parents from hell', who, as in so many authoritarian governments, didn't think I needed to know quite what would happen next. That was hardly surprising, when I think about it, as I was only too aware that the violent acts promoted by the goblins, whatever they might assert, would be disastrous for everybody including me. There would be no triumphant and responsibility-free, horror movie madness, showing me feasting on the evil power of babies and living forever. Or whatever.

Jealousy alone, however, can't really explain how all babies became classified as 'evil' and deserving of violent ends. Was I a violent and angry child? Well yes, sometimes. I have to admit to hitting or shoving a sibling during heated arguments but I never managed to inflict any more than transient pain. Luckily, the only weapons I used were my hands. Physical chastisement by adults was normal when I was growing up, so hitting siblings, while definitely wrong, wasn't as socially unacceptable as it might be today. Importantly, on a couple of occasions, teenage me learnt that 'seeing red' was an actual physiological state: I really could see nothing but a scorching hot, red wall of fury. These were the only times in life that I've ever truly seen red and it was during sibling rows. I can't remember the details, but I think my siblings were teasing me. Where did that anger go? I didn't see myself as an angry or violent adult; I never hit anybody, or had any desire to, and I had little interest in violent films or sport. Physical violence wasn't part of my conscious adult composition, but the anger is obviously there within me, even if it is rarely expressed - the goblins were an angry bunch.

I also remember having low level violent thoughts towards a baby brother. I wasn't really, considering the size of the family, overly burdened by childcare but he would sometimes be under my care while my mother was busy. It's possible, at some instinctive level, he sensed my hostility (or it may have been little more than me not giving him enough attention) as he would cry, loudly and constantly; he was a fine, vigorous baby. I don't remember feeling shocked by these mildly violent thoughts, although I knew they were wrong and felt somewhat unclean. At the time, I felt they were vaguely defensible. 'I'm trying to learn my French vocab, how many of my classmates have got to do this while trying to wind a stupid baby?'

The idea that these thoughts could take on a life of their own and actually hurt someone, independently of me, never crossed my mind. Disturbingly, I was saner at twelve than I was twenty years later. I knew these were just thoughts and no more than that. They didn't make me an evil person, particularly as I felt no compulsion, or even real desire, to act on them. There was no way that hurting a baby, for any reason other than necessary care (such as vaccinations), was justifiable in any context. There was also no sinister denouement to this story to feed my later paranoia and obsessional thinking. This particular baby grew up normally and is now a healthy, happily married father with a good job.

Going back further, into the bits I don't remember at all, it gets murkier. People trying to help me have focussed on trauma in my early years because, apart from the normal traumas of growing up such as the death of grandparents, this is the only other youthful trauma that I experienced. There are good reasons underpinning their search. Childhood trauma has often been implicated in the development of schizophrenia. It may cause abnormalities in the production of cortisol in the brain, leading to decreased stress tolerance and greater vulnerability to mental illness. Whether or not this explains my infanticidal desires is, yet again, only speculation.

I was my parents' first born, and a year or so later they had a healthy boy, who died suddenly and inexplicably from cot death. I can only imagine how my parents felt; my poor mother never mentioned the lost baby at all. It was all too traumatic. She did, however, keep a black and white photograph of him on her bedside table but, as we hardly went in my parents' bedroom, we wouldn't have known quite which one of us it was. Everything else, the letters, photos, and all the rest, was boxed up and for many years stored in the garage. My father didn't revisit this box until after my mother's death, a few years ago. Everybody's lives at that point - the tiny dead child, my parents, and me - were walled off, both literally and metaphorically.

As a result of this sudden tragedy, I was sent to stay with grandparents a long way from home. I wouldn't have known them that well and it was for several months, so quite a long period. There I was adored, to the extent that when I went home, my grandmother refused to clean off a muddy handprint I'd left on a door.

It's clear, at the very best, I would have received inconsistent emotional care during this period and probably some degree of maternal, emotional deprivation. My mother was deeply depressed by her son's death, which is why I stayed with my grandparents for so long. She was naturally a conscientious and anxious person and I'm sure she met my physical needs on my return. She would have done her best for me emotionally too, but the circumstances were horrible.

My father tells me her GP encouraged her to have another child, to help with her depression and, when she did, things became easier and normal life resumed. After this, my parents went on to have five more children; this was the lost little boy's tangible legacy, as they'd never intended to have a large family. My father describes it as 'substitute babies', to the extent the next boy shared his name with his dead brother. As each baby survived three months, my parents were looking for the next one, so a new baby was an especially happy, celebrative event. Therefore, killing a baby, any baby, was unsurprisingly, the absolutely worst thing I could possibly do - probably in any situation, but it would be particularly dreadful in our family.

Looking back, this tragedy affected all of our upbringings, although somewhat obliquely. My mother frequently assured us that babies and toddlers are supremely adaptable, in order to survive. She implied that the very young don't remember, or rather register, emotional trauma. As she was my mother, and had a number of children, I accepted this viewpoint, although I did wonder. I don't criticise her for teaching us this as I recognise her underlying pain and anxiety however, as a result, I didn't mention the baby's death, or my subsequent stays away from home, to anyone in mental health services for years.

Is this story relevant? It may or may not be, who's to say. It's a difficult area altogether as it's not my tragedy. I was only collateral damage and laying claim to that damage is an uncomfortable feeling. It feels like attention seeking and, even worse, attention seeking well after the event when everybody else had, to the best of their abilities, moved on.

A psychiatric nurse, trying to help me in later years, asked me to address my inner child directly. This was very difficult. What child? Where is she? She leaves no reliably identifiable traces in my consciousness, although she's presumably embedded in my brain. She's hardly a discrete person, and is probably no more than a bunch of feelings, some of which might emanate from her while others are probably nothing to do with her. All will have been edited over time. I can look at old photos of her and she looks quite sweet, but I can't reach out and touch her, not physically or emotionally. That child in the photos is no more than a one- dimensional doll, an arrangement of faded, coloured inks.

Practically speaking, how do you explain what's going on to a toddler? When I've babysat young relatives (not babies), while their parents go out for the day, the best I can do to alleviate their distress is to hug them, while repeatedly saying, 'Don't worry, mummy, daddy back soon.' Nobody could have reassured me this way, at least not truthfully.

What emotions did I have? Who knows. Small children are often jealous of an infant sibling. Did I blame him for the sudden separation and my mother's later depression? Did I get my mother back after the depression, only to lose her again when my sister was born? Did I end up investing all babies with the erroneous belief that they were very powerful and to be feared? That babies could pick me up and banish me? Or that they were surrounded by massive, unmanageable anxiety and could be all too easily harmed? To what extent did I think I was responsible for my suddenly upset life? The worst scenario of all, is, was this really a cot death tragedy or was I responsible for the death of this child? That, through the goblins, I'm just reliving something I've done already?

I'll never know, because the one person who was there (my father was at work) was too traumatised to talk about it, and I fully respected her privacy. I've never regretted not asking her, and now it's too late anyway. If she were still alive, I wouldn't be writing this book. In later years, we had a perfectly normal, loving relationship but I do have a troublesome fragment of memory, from when I was about five. She was leaning over me to kiss me goodnight, and I thought: 'Don't kiss me, I don't want you to, just go away.' Was this a reflection of a damaged bond? Or is it no more than a simple, meaningless childhood recollection? After all, there's no helpful context. Perhaps we'd had a row, or I'd been scolded for something or other.

As for that inner child? That's a psychoanalytic can of worms. To be honest, part of me is angry with her ... if ... if ... she exists somewhere or other. Would I really want to talk to her, even if I could? Look what she's done to me. If I wanted to kill an infant I'd choose her. I know how this child feels isn't her fault, but did she really rise up and destroy my life? Was she driving the goblins? Is she a goblin squatting in my brain? Both are hugely egocentric, in the way a small child has to be to survive. I want her, at the very least, safely locked in her box in the brain storage section marked: 'Unfortunate, get over it.' We all have this section, but mine appears to be uncomfortably porous.

Sadly, the goblins' destructive commands didn't stop when I moved south. In fact they upped the ante as I now had free access to an infant niece, in a nearby town, and my family had no idea the goblins wanted her dead, whatever the consequences. As ever, the goblins never bothered to address disastrous outcomes. I tried to avoid being alone with my niece because I knew I was an unsafe carer, but it was difficult. She was my own flesh and blood. Every bit of me yearned to be with her, but there was always goblin hate crawling, like lice, through my brain.

It came to a head one afternoon when I was asked to take her out by myself. Her mother needed a break and had things to do. It was an everyday sort of request - a fond auntie to mind the baby for a bit. It was the kind of situation I'd previously responsibly avoided, but my sister caught me off guard, and I wasn't brave or ethical enough to refuse. I couldn't resist the temptation; this child wasn't mine but I could pretend she was. I was never going to have a child of my own but people would think she belonged to me, or failing that, at least I was trusted enough to have sole charge of this precious little life.

When I took her out in the pushchair, all I could see of her were her tiny fat feet, kicking a little. All I heard from her were a few fragments of droning song and the odd random exclamation, which had me leaning over the pram hood and asking rhetorically, 'All right, poppet?' While she was awake she was safe, my attention was on her, but then she fell asleep and my attention wandered. It was a warm, overcast day. We walked around the local streets and then we went to the park. If she woke up, I thought, she could look at the birds on the large pond. I could also walk freely without worrying about potentially dangerous traffic.

As we approached the pond, I was coldly gripped by the strongest goblin compulsion I'd ever experienced. I knew that I'd erred all along, that she would have been safer at home, and here was the truth. How dare I take her out and risk her life. 'Drown her,' the goblins said. 'Drown her,' over, and over again. I gazed at the opaque still water and, in my mind's eye, watched the bubbles curling up from her mouth and her fine baby hair fanning out like pondweed. It was a quiet weekday afternoon, nobody was nearby or even looking in my direction. I could slide her out of the pushchair and, from that distance, nobody would realise it was empty. Everything, as I stood there, was hyper real, with the crisp soulless appearance of an old glass negative. It was as though I was no longer part of the physical world at all. The background noises were dissonant and fragmented, no longer forming a steady backdrop of the life of the town. I knew this feeling; it was shock. The goblins wanted to destroy her, destroy my family and destroy me.

No, I didn't drown her. I turned around and took her home. She was safe, totally unharmed, and as perfect as when I took her out. I knew I couldn't hurt her as I loved her too much, but the goblins easily could. I was appalled at the risk I had so arrogantly taken, even though I knew I myself was innocent of all these horrible ideas. After all, I'd known all along that I wouldn't get away with an untroubled saunter with the pram, hadn't I? What possessed me to go and look at the water? She wasn't going to wake up and enjoy the birds before we got home.

Had the goblins led me there? If so, drowning was a new venture for them.

Looking back, it's easy for me to say: 'Oh, underneath, I knew right from the beginning that the goblins weren't real and that it was really me who had unwanted thoughts about killing babies.' Those are the kind of intrusive thoughts and feelings that can underlie severe, distressing, obsessive compulsive disorder, but the OCD sufferer, I believe, accepts that their violent thoughts emanate from them. It's a version of events any sensible person would prefer because, while it must be difficult to live with, at least it's honest. The aberrant feelings can be unpicked and examined. However, it was almost impossible to argue with someone like me, who refused to even consider the core of the dispute. I should know how hard it is for people; I've blocked them at every turn. Surely, I can't have been so mad and stupid to have been taken in by the goblins' incredibly flimsy construction. I must have been a victim of calculated deceit. At least, that's what I like to think, but, in reality, the only fraudster was me. Flimsy or not, I stuck with this fraud for years, in spite of quantities of evidence to the contrary. I know this from my emotional reaction to finally accepting the truth - well, a distorted version of the truth - after being told so many, many times that I was wrong.

My family was paying for me to see the psychologist, Dr A, at the time, who finally, very, very forcibly, made me accept the violent thoughts as ... sort of ... my own. I was the goblins, the goblins were me, I wanted the child dead. But I also think my genuine love for the child also finally unlocked the truth in my brain. That insignificant afternoon, when I took my tiny niece out for an airing, was one of the worst days of my life. All the other threatened babies were, without saying, incredibly precious to their families and friends, but not incredibly precious to me. This baby was different.

It was a seismic shock. That evening, after the psychologist's appointment, I went home and tried to kill myself before giving up at 1am, tearful and exhausted. I went to bed and then went to work the following day. Life went on. I've never tried to commit suicide again. If I couldn't kill myself out of love, and the need to protect this child, I was never going to.

Meanwhile, NHS mental health services were left to pick up the pieces. As ever, I'd shared this unhappy story with them, while barely considering its impact and potential ramifications. My poor sister was called in and interviewed, by the then consultant, and warned that my access to the child must be strictly limited, otherwise social services would be involved. I thought this might wreck my relationship with my sister, but actually she was so angry that anyone could doubt her motherly instincts, i.e. that I was a safe carer for her daughter, that it brought us closer together. This was a huge relief to me as it implied, just about, that perhaps ... perhaps ... the goblins weren't as evilly omnipotent as I feared. Maybe, my family considered them unfortunate but manageable, even if I didn't.

This sad incident makes me think of the toxic ripples of my disease, and how they spread out and hurt so many innocent people: the good friend, an already anxious new mother; the manager at work, wondering how to reconcile an obviously psychotic employee with a responsible job that was based on caring, caring for inanimate objects, but caring nonetheless; my loving family, suddenly having to rescue an adult daughter they thought was managing fine, knowing she'd never be fully the same again and wondering quite what they'd done wrong; my sister, sitting in a consultant psychiatrist's office, being told who, and who couldn't, see her own daughter. The list goes on. How much I feel for them now, and so much for my sister. She was me five years before, furiously and unhappily discovering the extent of mental health service's legal powers.

I'd like to say that, after the psychologist's window-opening episode, I fully accepted the unreality of the goblins and was able to triumphantly embrace the long view but, to be honest, everything stayed very muddled. I stopped seeing that psychologist shortly afterwards, so he never really followed up the groundbreaking shift in my thinking. I was now working full time, and that was my priority. For the record, that year or so with the psychologist has been the only time I've used private healthcare.

So, it was only a partially-realised victory over the goblins and difficult to explain. Yes, the thoughts might be mine, but the goblins still wanted me to do terrible things. They still had a presence outside me. I, however, now saw myself as doubly dangerous and stinkingly corrupt. I had two drivers, my evil and the goblins' evil. It poisoned my system. I could feel black filaments pulsing through every limb in my body, spreading like mould through my arteries, veins, and capillaries. This evil was frighteningly alive. I'd always known I had great potential for evil - the goblins wouldn't have chosen me otherwise - but this was confirmation of this horrible truth, and it was a lot worse than I'd thought. Any claims to my relative innocence, however shaky, were gone forever. I was racked with guilt and self-loathing.

I worried incessantly about the harm I could do to my niece, just by being near her, as though the evil would somehow spread from me and infect her innocent soul. She might be physically unwell or spiritually damaged; the possibilities were endless. I was always watching and hoping she'd be OK. I felt like a wicked fairy godmother, hovering malignly round the crib with my unholy goblin assistants.

I could not even begin to consider the ancient conundrum: does having evil thoughts make you an evil person? I was a million miles from that sane twelve year old. To be honest, if I look at the issue dispassionately (which can be difficult), the answer is, 'of course not.' Everyone has thoughts they'd rather not have, although mine can be nastier than many; if there's a hierarchy of 'bad' thoughts, baby killing must be well towards the top. However, I've never actually acted on any of the 'bad' thoughts. For example, the museum where I worked really doesn't have a history of unexplained fires. At the time, I was so enmired in poisonous guilt, I couldn't grasp this distinction at all; my words and deeds were all mixed up together. This made me very difficult to deal with because I would take on the emotional turmoil of the evil deed, even if I hadn't actually committed it.

And was my little niece damaged, in any way at all? If she was, it's not obvious. She's almost grown up now, and she's healthy, intelligent and beautiful. So are all my other nephews and nieces. At time of writing, the youngest is a baby.

Baby killing desires and feelings were never so strong again, but they still formed an unwelcome backdrop to my life for years, waxing and waning in intensity in line with my mental health. That niece has been followed by more nephews and nieces, so my existence has been complicated by a line of potential little victims, but my infanticidal desire has been emasculated by frequent unfulfilled reruns, rather like my desire for suicide. I didn't kill the child then, so I'm unlikely to kill a child now. It's more like the 'polar bear' theory these days. I dance a baby up and down on my knee, while part of me is thinking, 'Whatever you do, just don't think about goblins.' So, of course I think about goblins as that, unfortunately, is how the brain works. It's best to keep the goblins right on the periphery of the action, shadowy and silent, even if I can't eliminate them altogether.

I've chosen not to have children of my own, although I would have loved to. All through my childhood, and into adulthood, I fantasised about my own future motherhood. I planned names in my school rough book when I was supposed to be paying attention in lessons but, thankfully, I was slow and shy when it came to baby making.

Once I developed psychosis, it was very unlikely I was going to have a child even if I achieved a long term, supportive relationship. My siblings have provided grandchildren so there was no familial pressure, and I gain infinite pleasure from being an aunt to my ready-made family. How lucky I am. More importantly, there is a genetic component to psychosis, so could I really bring up a child knowing their life might unfold like mine? I would be waiting, watching, ever anxious. How could I play roulette with someone I loved? As far as I'm concerned, this is the upside of eugenics. After all, eugenics can be positive if you're the one making the decisions.

In addition, my pregnancy and onwards would be stalked by psychiatrists, social workers and an anguished and conflicted family. It would hardly be a happy start for the little one. Neither could I promise ongoing mental stability as a mother. Would my child be emotionally, and intellectually, stymied by having to be my carer? Worst of all, would I have ended up actually creating a victim of my own, especially for the goblins?

The only 'children' I have now are those that occasionally appear in my dreams. Not daydreams, but rather the dreams we have at night, when all sorts of bits of pieces float to the surface. I am never a violent mother there but, instead, I'm profoundly neglectful. When did I last feed my baby? (Gender unspecified, the sad little mite never has a name.) I'm not sure. I was busy doing other things and the poor baby was wilfully forgotten by me. I gaze at it fearfully. Is it still alive? Or, perhaps, I've let my baby get too cold. I'm dressed warmly but the poor baby is almost naked under a thin summer blanket. This frozen baby always looks particularly dead; the little wax doll I'd read about in literature, rather like the imitation real-life baby dolls that desperate, maternally-thwarted women buy. After all, for all my threats, I've never actually seen a dead baby in real life, only my dead mother.

Then there's the million dollar question. Am I still a dangerous person? The answer, sadly, is yes, especially if I don't take antipsychotic medication. The baby killing pathways have been laid down and reinforced in my neural circuits. There are underlying miswirings in my brain. Antipsychotic medication helps me manage these weird wirings, and focus on the more normal, and fulfilling, aspects of life, but it doesn't fix the underlying issues. I'm relying on a safety net of medication, family, friends, society's expectations, the inevitable ghastly aftermath of infanticide; extraordinary distress all round, retribution and incarceration, lifelong guilt and all the rest.

However, there's a big problem. I don't know when I'm going to be psychotic again and what form it might take. Back in 1998, if you'd told me I was going to be psychotically ill,
I would have been extremely startled and frightened, but it would have been, just about, within the bounds of probability. Had you then added that I would, for years, be controlled by malevolent goblins, that appeared to be pretty much unique to me, I would have laughed incredulously, wondered about your sanity, and then concluded that I must have misheard you.

I have, occasionally, been temporarily removed from society under mental health laws, but my ongoing liberty has been underwritten by a society that generally believes it is wrong to punish on the basis of potential criminality, rather than actual criminality. In a less liberal society, I could be locked away long term. In Hitler's Germany, I would be dead. Would that be the safest option for those around me? Have my baby killing desires really been worked through? What if a future delusional world, yet again, includes baby killings? What if the goblins were only a friendly warm up act? There's obviously no logic to my choice of delusion. Next time, the command hallucinations could be stronger.

I like to think not. I like to think that the powerful negative emotions that drove me will never be as powerful and controlling again. But I don't know. Nobody does. That's the problem.

CHAPTER 16 AFTERMATH

My story doesn't end in spring 2002. The person I was then could hardly be writing this now. I don't have copies of my medical notes after I left that northern town, so it's mostly down to my sometimes unreliable memory and some later clinic letters. There's nothing legally to stop me requesting them and, apart from my very good GP, most of the people I've had dealings with have moved on in their careers. Even so, I do encounter them occasionally on the High Street and watch them run for cover. It's wryly amusing. Do they think I'm going to bore on about my mental health? I do know what the boundaries are. Therefore, I'd really rather not know what they've written about me. Equally, these days, most of the psychiatric nurses and other mental health staff are younger than me and still working, so I have to be careful what I write. I don't want to damage someone's career, however inadvertently. It's a minefield. I'm talking about real people here, not goblins.

When I left the northern town, I was convinced it was the end - the end of everything.There was no sense of relief, just abject failure. It would be a couple of years before I realised how privileged I was to be offered a fresh start; a fresh start that I hadn't earned in any way. I just got lucky.

I was emotionally wrecked. For years, the name of the town I'd just left was so painful I couldn't bear it in any context; as a person's surname, as a street name or district in another part of the country. It was, after all, the principal home of the all-powerful goblins, whose life-destroying predictions had come true in spite of everyone's reassurances.

I'd been told time and time again that the goblins were imaginary constructs of my illness, but here they were validated by cold, hard circumstances. They were real, they were powerful and they'd won. Everything I'd worked so hard for was gone. It was an important lesson; if you play with fire, you end up burnt. In some ways I had, for over two years, been playing. In spite of all those goblin threats, I'd still had my house and, even though I was off sick, I still had my job and therefore my career. Now I didn't, the game was over and I had to live with the consequences.

Yet again, I was knowingly running at least two narratives simultaneously. Version one, was that the goblins had selected me as their submissive evil partner and had, possibly as a result of my disobedience (lack of dead babies, in particular), destroyed my life. Version two, was that it was all the fault of the museum. After all, unlike many schizophrenics, I didn't run into trouble until I was thirty. I'd been resilient enough to cope with examinations and moving around the country in my teens and twenties, therefore it must be the museum that had caused this mess. Somewhere deep down, I hope, there must have been a version three, which would have been that it wasn't the museum's fault per se, but it was my reaction to the museum and my new life that was the problem. However, I'm not sure at that time I was capable of this rather more accurate reading of the situation. Version four, which lurked unacknowledged and even deeper down, was that a combination of genes and upbringing had left me a ticking time bomb, more vulnerable to ordinary stress than many.

The museum world is small and even though I continued with museum voluntary work, sporadically for several years, it was increasingly clear to me that I would never again work as a specialist curator. Crucially, I knew I'd never even have an opportunity to go back. Even if I did manage to convince someone I was a safe bet (highly unlikely), it would probably mean moving somewhere else, and my days of confidently moving round the country were over. I mourned my museum career and missed the prestige. The museum world was quite competitive and I'd done respectably well to end up where I had. It was an attention-attracting job as there aren't that many museum curators. I'd also genuinely liked my colleagues, largely because they were not only really nice people, but because we shared similar interests and backgrounds.

I still dream at night, though less so now, about this amputation. My manager is always in this dream; she's re-appointed me, but the other details are sketchy and variable, apart from the enormous sense of relief I feel. Then I wake up and I'm briefly, catastrophically scared. I haven't got a home and I haven't got a job ... and then? It's twenty years ago, I suddenly realise, so stop panicking, everything's moved on. You don't have to start rebuilding your life.

This loss of career was also a major blow to my sense of self. My personal interests and my career had been tightly enmeshed. I love antiques, art, country houses, living history, redundant factories and all the rest of Britain's (and the world's) extensive heritage. My museum jobs gave me a chance to share this enthusiasm and to help look after our nation's history. I wanted people to understand and enjoy this as much as I did. If I could make people happy and educate them at the same time, I would be happy too. It wasn't a very noble ambition, after all heritage is fairly far down in the list of life's essentials, but it felt better than trying to sell mobile phone contracts. Now, I was totally shut out of this world, not only professionally, but personally. All this wonderful, life-affirming heritage, was to me at this time, little more than a heap of junk. It would take several years of cautious experiments before I would rediscover this pleasure.

Now, I'm reasonably glad I don't work in a museum anymore, as there's no professional pressure. I don't have to realise big projects over months; liaise with people such as the press when I am feeling shy; research and publish; and let museums eat up my spare time: the working day is no longer elastic. But I'll never lose my museum curator identity totally. When I visit galleries, exhibitions and museums, I'm still looking at how the display was realised - the lighting, the stands, the interpretation boards. Never mind the exhibits themselves. In fact I'm cross on both the exhibits' and the visitors' behalf if I think the curators have let them down. I know exactly how much hard work is needed to mount a good exhibition, or a good permanent display.

Finally, for all my nostalgia for the museum world, I have to admit that my brain is irrevocably damaged. I'm in the difficult situation of having the qualifications, but no longer the necessary intellect. I've assiduously practised concentration for years and years but it's never fully recovered, and that's just the surface of the mental flexibility I've lost, along with other skills. My family would have supported me going back into education to take a further degree but, sadly, there was no chance of that.

With my father at work, my mother took the brunt of my rehabilitation. It was incredibly tough for her. She was having to deal every day with a tearful, hopeless daughter. Day in, day out, I was dreary, unfocussed, ungiving and irritable, and always hanging about or lying awake in bed. I rarely went out by myself and generally showed little interest or enthusiasm when I was taken anywhere, even when the visits were clearly designed as treats for me. I soaked up support from my parents and siblings and was unable to give anything back. I was the human equivalent of a black hole.

Frustratingly for my parents, trying to rationalise goblins with me was a total dead end and the issue was rarely explored. It wasn't because they didn't want to help me, but more that they didn't know how. They researched psychosis, primarily to help me, but also to help themselves: how to deal with me and, most importantly, how to free themselves from the accusatory shadow of R D Laing. Of course, my upbringing wasn't perfect, nobody's is, but my parents genuinely tried their best. So, I'm relieved they dismissed Laing and his, inadvertently cruel, and now outdated theory that, 'it's all the fault of the parents.' My mother and father had enough to deal with, poor things, and they always looked embarrassed and uncomfortable if goblins were mentioned. I remember David Icke and the giant lizards being rolled out for my contemplation, but I couldn't see what that had to do with goblins at all. After all, giant lizards are patently ridiculous, aren't they? Who would believe in them? Crucially, why is laughing at giant lizards the same as laughing at goblins? Somewhere around this point they gave up, evidently concluding that a better approach would be to bolster my normal, functioning side and then, hopefully, the goblins would subside and I'd be able to resume a more normal life.

For the first three months or so, I had no external medical support and this exacerbated my family's problems. Before moving I had been receiving quite intensive intervention, where the next step would have been hospital admission. As a result, the goblins remained largely unaired and festered horribly. The only medical professional I saw was my new GP, to ensure the continuation of my prescription. Looking back, I probably should have explained the situation to her and she could have acted as my intermediary. I didn't realise she would do that (she has subsequently done so, very effectively) as she had told me that in this new, larger practice, the GPs usually divided the specialities up between them and hers wasn't mental health. This complicated our relationship for years and years, as although I generally liked and trusted her (and was nervous of the other GPs), I rarely came clean about mental health issues, as I believed I wasn't supposed to discuss them with her.

I've included this example, as it shows how capable I was of taking one observation - not a prohibition - from 2002, and building a whole, negative delusional structure around it. The belief I'm 'not supposed' to talk to my new GP developed into a goblin-endorsed: 'I'm not allowed'. Who said I wasn't? Me or the GP? She never used such concrete terms and I definitely wasn't forbidden from her consulting room unless I produced the right kind of disorder. It was all down to me and my anxious feelings which then, unsurprisingly, were incorporated into negative goblin lore ... I can trace it through. Now I don't worry about goblins; I am 'allowed' to speak openly to my GP about mental health, which is helpful.

Eventually, after some complaining (to the previous mental

health service), I saw various psychiatric nurses, although it would be a while until there was any stability there. I also received an appointment with a psychiatrist. Off we went again. The psychiatrist decided to prescribe clozapine again, this time off-label, with the addition of lithium as it increases the white blood cell count. Thanks to this lithium prescription, I would spend the next couple of years explaining to medical and semi-medical types that, no, I wasn't bipolar and, no, they needn't be alert to manic episodes.

It was back to hospital again, but on very different terms this time; it was purely so clozapine could be initiated. This new psychiatric ward (which is long closed and local mental health services are now run by another trust) provided an alarming and uncomfortable environment. There was only one tiny positive; it had a small amount of secure, outside space. For the first time, I was sharing my living space with disturbed, potentially dangerous (at least that's how it felt), unwashed young men. Their general grubbiness was unsurprising; the washing facilities and ward were very dirty, and few members of staff bothered to see that patients got up at a reasonable time, washed, or ate at mealtimes. The food was dreadful, so a lot of patients relied on supplies provided by their visitors. Most of the staff, mainly male student nurses (I can't remember any female nursing staff at all), appeared to resent any interruption by the lowly hopeless (i.e. us, the patients) and rarely ventured further than the glass box by the ward front door, which meant, as the ward was an odd shape, parts of it appeared totally unmonitored. I actually felt some nostalgia for that northern hospital, which was suddenly no longer the worst place in my experienced world. However, this new ward was bearable as I knew that my admission was for two weeks only and there was, thankfully, an agreed release date.

For the first few weeks I had clozapine-induced nausea again, caused by low blood pressure. Fortunately, nobody at the hospital noticed, but my mother, somewhat embarrassed, became used to hanging around various public places when we were out together. I would crouch on the floor, with my head between my knees telling her it was fine, nothing sinister and it would pass, so we just got on with it.

There was, however, another more troublesome side effect. This time, clozapine gave me mild epilepsy which was, initially, limited to myoclonic jerks (I spilled a lot of tea) during the morning. It felt as though someone had flicked a switch in my brain: on, off, on. My mother would look at me and say:

'There, you've done it again. Why do you keep doing that?' in a slightly exasperated manner. I think she thought it was some kind of nervous tic, which I'd occasionally suffered from in childhood. I didn't know what it was except that, unlike with tics, there was no building sense of compulsion, no battle for suppression. These 'jumps', or whatever they were, just happened. There was no way I could control them.

Later, I started falling to my knees as well and, occasionally, would find myself flat on my face with no recollection of how I got there. I remember a chap leaping out of his car near Sainsbury's and shouting:

'Are you all right?!'

'Yes, I'm fine, thanks,' I replied, while thinking, 'Oh, marvellous ...'

It was true, I was fine. I never hurt myself, I'd just go floppy. The lack of any warning at all was the worst problem (unlike the low blood pressure) but, luckily, it never happened at the top of a flight of steps.

'Don't hold my arm!' I'd forcibly tell my mother, having alarming visions of her falling down the steps with me, but a mother is a mother and I think she found it difficult to resist.

This particular side effect was a totally new experience for me, but I was so indifferent to anything other than my grief at losing my former life that I don't remember being particularly concerned. It just goes to show how demoralised I was. I'm sure that before my illness, I'd have been extremely alarmed if I were collapsing in the street without any warning, and with no understanding as to why, but now it was ... whatever. The myoclonic jerks had been picked up on the ward by a junior doctor. This was by observation, as there was no way I was going to complain about anything that might prolong my admission. She'd prescribed an anti-Parkinson's medication, probably procyclidine which I'd had before, as involuntary movements can be a side effect of antipsychotics, especially the older ones.

At my next outpatient appointment, safely out of hospital by now, I mentioned this unfamiliar problem, a problem that had deeply concerned my family, though not me. The consultant said, consideringly, 'Hmm, perhaps we should try a different approach and see if that helps.' About a year later, when working temporarily in the local NHS occupational health department, I illicitly read my file and found the 'hmm, perhaps ...' expressed much more strongly to my GP, along the lines of, 'I have absolutely no idea why she was prescribed this as it would have done her no good whatsoever.' He was right, his anti-epileptic prescription, sodium valproate, fixed the problem. This particular medication has been linked with birth defects but, for the record, unlike many women, I was warned about this at the time.

I stayed on clozapine for a couple of years and then I stopped it when I was under mental duress - basically after endangering my niece's life in the park - and reverted to my bad, old, medication-denying habits. This was not through lack of insight when it came to my illness; it was a deliberate act of self-harm to mitigate my guilty feelings. Perhaps also, I felt betrayed by the medication and was pushing it away metaphorically, while saying, 'It doesn't work, it didn't protect the precious child. So, what's the point of taking it?' Mixed emotions, as ever.

After a certain amount of to-ing and fro-ing, I ended up on quetiapine which I still take. Clozapine has been mentioned subsequently by psychiatrists, but has never been prescribed for me again because of the side effects. I think I might have stopped quetiapine a couple of times near the beginning, but I've never stopped it fully since, although I have sometimes reduced the dose - not to good effect when I've gone too far. Whatever my dreams, hopes and desires, I have eventually learnt that I, personally, need to take antipsychotic medication, but I'd still rather I didn't have to.

In about 2005, my diagnosis was changed to schizoaffective disorder. As I have never been manic, I guess it's the depressive variety. I was, to my surprise, sorry to lose the schizophrenia label, as it was a label that had been incorporated, however uncomfortably, into my identity. The 'labelling' of mental health patients is, for some, a hugely controversial area but being 'labelled' doesn't bother me. In fact I prefer it, as I know where I am, and anyway my diagnostic label is only one small part of my overall composition. I missed the schizophrenia label, as everyone, including me, knows that schizophrenia is a severe mental illness, and I could use it as a cover for all sorts of uncomfortable feelings and failures.

Back in 2005 or thereabouts, a schizoaffective disorder diagnosis was more nebulous. Some professionals disputed its existence as a separate condition at all, an opinion that I, particularly in darker moods, would deliberately misinterpret. 'I've got an illness that doesn't exist, therefore I'm malingering,' I'd say to myself, wilfully ignoring the fact that the professionals who doubted schizoaffective disorder's existence preferred to describe its sufferers as either 'schizophrenic' or 'bipolar'.

Even now, at time of writing, the NHS A-Z website of health conditions does not have a dedicated schizoaffective disorder section and schizoaffective disorder only appears, as it sometimes does, as a 'not schizophrenia' note in the schizophrenia pages. 'Not schizophrenia', is an odd diagnosis to have, especially as the NHS has separate pages for other mental health problems, such as body dysmorphic disorder and seasonal affective disorder.

Ah yes, seasonal affective disorder ... Some, usually American, writers have, in the past, used the acronym SAD for schizoaffective disorder. However, in the UK, SAD is usually used for seasonal affective disorder, a winter depression brought on by lessening daylight hours. I was worried, particularly when unable to work, that occupational health and management would think I had the latter, rather less problematic condition, and would be hoping my problems could, at least partially, be resolved by sitting under a daylight bulb. That said, perhaps I shouldn't be so dismissive; maybe a daylight bulb might be helpful, as the goblins have always preferred long dark evenings.

Thus, it was my usual paradoxical black and white thinking. 'I have a serious, chronic mental illness,' or 'I'm malingering,' with not much in between. It largely depended on my varying state of mind and who I was dealing with. The last word goes to my mother, who said that, as far she was concerned, this 'schizoaffective disorder thing' appeared to be the same as what I'd had all along.

However, my new, somewhat unwanted diagnosis turned out to be unexpectedly valuable. For the first time, since the month's trial of antidepressants shortly after my initial referral to mental health services, I was prescribed antidepressants alongside the antipsychotic medication. I've been taking them on and off ever since and they are very helpful. My negative, ambushing emotions are under better control, so I'm less paranoid and anxious. This means that I feel generally more able to cope with life and, as a result, am braver. I don't think I would be writing this now, if I wasn't taking antidepressants.

Meanwhile, my parents were busy sorting me out. This was a humiliating experience but necessary; left to my own devices I would have just drifted. We combined resources and I ended up with my own home, closer to the family, in the southern town where I'd grown up. House prices are high down here and I never forget how lucky I am. My kind and supportive parents wanted me to have a roof over my head, whatever happened.

After a couple of years my parents retired to the seaside partly (but only partly) because I'd worn out my poor mother. I'm not surprised, as she had really tried to support and encourage me and, much as I loved her, I have to admit that she didn't really have the right kind of temperament for nursing, either physical or mental. (Neither do I.) I remember her saying crossly, on one occasion, that it seemed to her that the goblins only stopped me from doing things I didn't want to do anyway. I thought this pronouncement was deeply unjust at the time, but now it makes me laugh.

I was left to sink or swim, but there was always the proviso that if I really did sink my parents would fish me out of troubled waters. I swam ... a bit haphazardly sometimes, but I managed to stay afloat. My mother telephoned me regularly and I had the support of nearby siblings. Best of all were the free holidays at the seaside, which I treasured. Walking along an almost empty sandy beach is, as so often observed, very good for mental health; the neutrality, the power of the water, the long view perspective, and all the rest.

There was the issue of employment. Again, I was pushed on by my parents, which was fine by me; I wasn't happy living on benefits. But what job could I do? The museum world was now closed to me and, while I was amply qualified to look after museum art collections, those skills weren't very transferable. Customer service or customer facing roles are a bit of an ordeal - for both me and my customer - though I can, and have worked with the public. I wasn't too keen on being a cleaner, my driving was, and is, terrible, and as for care work ... vulnerable people of any age would be natural goblin targets, so that was one hundred percent a bad idea.

That left clerical work and that's where I started, as a NHS clerical volunteer. With the encouragement of my new supervisor this led to temporary, paid work and finally, thankfully, a full time permanent job in medical records at the local hospital. It was hardly exciting or glamorous and the pay was less than I'd earned in museums, but I was so grateful to my new NHS employers. Who else would have wanted me? I hadn't succeeded in convincing the NHS to take me on (I tried) until I'd been doing the job as a temporary staff member for nearly a year. My CV was extremely suspicious, not because I lied, but

I was, for starters, obviously over-qualified. Had I got further, that occupational health file on me which I'd illicitly read, stated that I should never be offered permanent NHS employment anyway. Not that this was ever mentioned to me. When I was finally offered the permanent NHS job, I was interviewed by the doctor who led the occupational health team; I was, clearly, still a dubious individual.

This is a good example of the stigma of mental illness. This isn't a memoir of how badly I've been treated (basically, I haven't) but, yes, of course I'm fully aware that my medical history affects how people perceive me. I remember going to the chemist to get my first antipsychotic prescription, and how the pharmacist looked at me with a degree of curiosity and, perhaps, compassion. It was the same look I'd received from the hospital phlebotomist earlier that day. Nobody, to my knowledge, had ever looked at me like that before. 'Well, that's strange,' I thought, not knowing why, and totally unaware that many more pharmacists and others were going to be looking at me the same way for years to come.

Then there are the dentists, who can't get me out of the chair fast enough. That's more of a positive actually, as I'm never pressured to have anything but the most basic and cheap dental care. Rather more annoying are the doctors' receptionists who engage with me, civilly and constructively, until they bring up my record and then suddenly physically and mentally recoil. Doctors' receptionists are famous for being difficult but I can usually time my difficulties to a second ... 'One, two, three ... she's read my grime screen ... yep, any attempt at a sensible conversation is now over. And no, I'm not considering bursting through your plastic window and throttling you ... whatever you're thinking.' That said, the opening summary box, in all my clinic letters, includes the words: 'Symptoms have included insomnia, feeling confused, paranoid and violent thoughts, suicidal ideas and delusions and hallucinations relating to goblins.' Would you trust this person? Possibly not.

Once I'd achieved a proper permanent job I could do, I clutched it like a life raft; you couldn't have prised away my fingers. I was proud to work for the NHS. It was a useful job, making sure that the right paperwork was in place for the doctors and nurses, and it was entirely clear that my contribution was an essential, if tiny, part of a patient's successful hospital stay or clinic visit. That was a good feeling, a very good feeling indeed.

Most importantly of all, the job slowly started to drag me out of my self-imposed hell. Suddenly, I was processing paperwork for people who could be in terrible situations, at worst facing death, and some of these unlucky souls were younger than me. Many had already endured a lifetime of chronic illness; others had been ambushed by illness out of the blue. What options did these people have? It made me think: 'Was what happened to me really such a disaster? How many of my apocalyptic goblin pronouncements have actually come true?' I was healthy and protected by my family, and I could now rebuild my life. Some poor patients had no opportunities left at all.

Practically speaking, the job suited me; at the end of each day I could walk away. My previous thoughts of workplace arson had evaporated; there wasn't much space now for nightmarish imaginings. I appreciated the non-negotiable deadlines and clear targets as they gave automatic shape and purpose to my day. There was little subjectivity involved, apart from how long you were prepared to look for errant paperwork. I quite enjoyed this bit, as it was a chance to think a little more creatively. I still hated making mistakes and would brood miserably and anxiously over my errors but, realistically speaking, they were never catastrophic. The paperwork I supplied had to be checked again by the nurse in the clinic, and then, finally, by the doctor. Yes, I would be reprimanded, but management would have to deal with the consequences and that would be the end of it. I was as careful as I could be because harming other people doesn't come naturally to me. Seriously? What about homicidal goblins?

Well, erm ... Luckily, the goblins were totally uninterested in hospital paperwork so any mistakes were firmly mine.

I got on reasonably well with my new colleagues - as usual I wanted a quiet life - so I was only rarely embroiled in internecine office wars. Unfortunately, some colleagues believed I thought myself better than them, which wasn't the case at all, unless they did a terrible job. At least I tried. Those people would have been surprised how much envious credit I gave them simply for achieving such basic, lifestyle desirables as finding a partner and having a family. Then there were those who thought me weird (fair enough), and there were a few occasions when people pointed out to me the futility of my university career, as I'd ended up in a job I could have got at sixteen. Well yes, in the circumstances, all that education was rather pointless. I didn't need people telling me that, although it did occur to me that many of my colleagues had paid for all that education via their taxes.

Could I have progressed a little, from the lowest NHS clerical pay band? Possibly, but it wasn't a question I wanted to ask. Far too risky. I earned enough for my quiet life and that was that. Work, even at this basic level, took a huge amount of effort, largely because it was tough keeping my thoughts straight all day and controlling my natural tendency to irrational paranoia when things were challenging. I eventually stayed with the medical records job until the end of 2020. I'd had three long absences over the years because of relapses. A private employer would have let me go, but the NHS kept me on. Another reason to be grateful.

My support from mental health services continued, and I met quite a number of psychiatric nurses over the next few years. Two of these spent longish periods working with me and were very good, both intelligent and engaged. One was a particularly kind and gentle young woman. At the time, I was very preoccupied and tearful, following the incident with my baby niece in the park, and obsessed by the evil running through my veins.

To my horror, this nurse was soon, very obviously, pregnant. Every time we met, the goblins expressed their usual dark desires, ordering me to stab her in the stomach and kill her 'evil' baby. I brought these sinister commands into the small clinic room with me, turning the room cold, with its institutional strip lighting and harshly black windows, shadowed by the winter dusk. But I said nothing at all about these goblin orders; the danger I brought in with me, although I felt guilty as hell. What an irresponsible coward I was, although I never brought a weapon to our meetings. But, surely, mental health services shouldn't have allowed a pregnant nurse to be in the same room as me? What were they thinking? It wasn't safe. In their defence, however, how much did they know about me? My new medical notes file was slim, so local services could access very little of my extensive history in the northern town; a history that recorded me wanting to stab my friend in the stomach and kill her 'evil' baby. Maybe, once the NHS is fully digitised, this dangerous lack of interface will be sorted out. I know, having just left a medical records job, that hospital files are still inaccessible to other hospital trusts, and rely on a secretary (usually), to send a selection of vital paperwork on - if requested. (Unlike the less comprehensive GP paper records, which do follow the patient.)

Certainly, this nurse's pregnancy added another layer of complication and stress to our meetings. I hope she didn't sense the goblin hostility; it was something she didn't deserve to know. This was something I felt at the time (and now), but truthfully speaking, that was a minor consideration. Of course I should have mentioned these goblin commands, but I was too ashamed and valued this nurse's input too much. By now I'd encountered several other psychiatric nurses, who were, perhaps, not entirely suited to this challenging job.

I'd seen one nurse, several times, who at each meeting did no more than read off the same list of questions of the strictly practical type:

'Are you sleeping? Are you taking your medication?' and all

the rest.

Tick, tick, tick down his form. His manner was about as cold and withdrawn as he could manage; there was no attempt at eye contact. I've had more personal interaction when talking to a building society. He made no attempt to quantify my thoughts, let alone offer me any support or ideas for dealing with them.

Another nurse spent our entire first interview swinging her foot and telling me it wasn't fair that she had so many patients. She then kept no further appointments, leaving me hanging about waiting for her. I got the message and buggered off, wondering why I was responsible for the local lack of mental health staffing. Because I was irresponsibly mad perhaps? A drain on society? It wasn't exactly a role in life I'd knowingly chosen for myself.

Worst of all, was a nurse who couldn't understand me and I, because I was brought up in the middle class south, have a reasonably neutral accent. I can tell this story, because I think he was an agency nurse, and his position in the local community mental health team was, unsurprisingly, fleeting. We met only once, a meeting that was entirely given over to an attempt to fill in a form with my personal details, but we ended up irrevocably jammed on the first line of my address, specifically the word 'View'. He got crosser and crosser as I kept offering to write it down. I don't know why he didn't accept this easy way out for both of us. Pride? Defensiveness? A fear of being found lacking, particularly when it came to his grasp of English? A strong preconception that as I was the loony one, I was officially the problem? A powerful desire to make me go away? (That worked).

I also wonder, while writing this now, quite what he thought I was saying? Did he think I was saying, 'avenue', and then refusing to accept it when he repeated it back to me? If that was the case, in my defence, our lack of understanding was already a two way problem. Or did he think I was saying 'you', as in 'you should know what my address is, it's recorded a multitude of times on your systems?' This, of course, was what I was thinking, and did suggest but definitely more politely. It might explain why he was annoyed; he thought I was being deliberately rude and, perhaps also, he thought I was consciously (or unconsciously) playing games? Which, of course, I wasn't; a psychiatric nurse might hope to help you abandon delusional ideas and all the rest, but this was my home address, so it wasn't really negotiable.

This all changed in about 2006, when I was extremely lucky (and by then, didn't I know it) to meet a psychiatric nurse (or rather, care co-ordinator as they are more often called today) who I would see on and off for the next ten years until she retired. During this period she discharged me twice. This was fine by me, although I was always anxious about it. When I ran into trouble she would pick up my case again. She was friendly, intelligent, persevering and cheerful, and with this steady, empathetic support I began, eventually, to drop my habitual defensiveness and unpick the goblin disaster. Importantly, she metaphorically took me by the hand and reassured me that whatever I might feel or believe about mental health services, they were there to help me and co-operating with them was a safe thing to do.

I'm not proud it took so long to accept this, as I'd hardly been treated badly. So, after all the years of war, or rather semi-war in later years, I finally approached mental health services with a reasonably open mind and generally positive attitude. They could actually be helpful, I discovered, especially when I listened to what they suggested, tried to follow through with their ideas, and even said thank you! After how long? This care co-ordinator also helped me to write things down about my illness. This was a big deal for me; people had been encouraging me to do this for years and I'd been too scared, as I thought writing things down confirmed and nourished the awfulness of the evil I engendered and surrounded myself with. It was a great leap forward, as having finally got over this deeply rooted fear, we all discovered that I was able to think things through when I write in a way I couldn't do in normal conversation.

In 2016, I also saw an NHS psychologist, and again tried to be as constructive as possible. My relationship with mental health services had definitely matured. It was increasingly difficult for me to be childishly defensive, when I was dealing with professionals many years younger than me. This psychologist was not quite fully qualified, but she was very competent, engaged and friendly, and I found myself feeling protective, even vaguely maternal towards her. Not that I remember telling her this - I didn't want to undermine her self confidence. As she was a trainee, I was expected to provide feedback on her performance, so I mentioned one small negative. The poor girl looked totally crestfallen. Oh dear ... However, these protective feelings encouraged me to be a 'good' patient so that she would take away some positivity from our meetings and would be able to consider me a success story. It was a win-win situation for both of us.

We discussed self-compassion and not being overly self-critical, which is probably a good thing, but it's tricky to achieve a balance when you're being asked to be clear eyed about your negative emotions and motivations. We examined my maladaptive coping mechanisms. I was encouraged to work things through, rather than run away and hope for the best, and also to accept that stress and anxiety were at the root of my issues. Mindfulness and deep breathing exercises, unsurprisingly, turned out to be a dead end. I could have told her that before we tried, as I was a child who didn't understand that breathing is an automatic process, and periodically worried that if I forgot to breathe, I might die.

So, I was able to draw on all this support and experience, and spent four years, totally successfully away from the community mental health team, dutifully taking the antipsychotic as prescribed. I felt quite proud of myself, thinking: 'This is it, I've finally cracked it, I'll never need mental services again.'

CHAPTER 17 AGAIN AND AGAIN?

I would like to say that when I moved back down south, my goblin love affair quietly ended, but no, we were to remain intimate until only a few years ago. While writing this I've had a quiet goblin companion or two, which is proof you can't eliminate them entirely. Predictably, they are hanging around in a slightly damp corner by the chimney breast in my Victorian house, their usual internal habitat. I can feel them watching me but that's as far as it goes. If I want to, I can summon them up elsewhere - I choose not to - but the chimney breast goblins appeared by themselves. I don't know if they would materialise if I moved to a relatively modern property but I'm not particularly worried by their company. They are no more than shadows.

Do I still believe in goblins? On balance not, but it's a difficult one. I've had many years of goblin belief and you can't just eliminate them from the brain's memory, emotional, visual, imagination and auditory circuits. Goblins are now hardwired in my brain. Intellectually, I can no longer support their reality, but I can only maintain this with a certain degree of mental discipline. As soon as a goblin thought comes up in my brain, I surreptitiously slip away into something, anything really, just not goblin. My chief concern is to stop reinforcing the old goblin circuits and, even more importantly, to not add new ideas to the belief structure. Without fresh ideas this belief system stagnates, becomes impoverished and is a less alluring, or rather less attention-demanding, place for me to visit.

Emotionally, it's more difficult as I have far less control over my emotions than my intellect. The goblin mythology feeds on negative emotion: on fear, anger, hate, anxiety and all the rest. Those emotions feel like a deep, dark pit inside. It's more difficult to turn off emotions like a tap; given half a chance they ambush and control. I can't stop the negative emotions we all have in daily life and they can trigger nihilistic, frightening, goblin-infested thoughts. Sometimes I might live with the revived goblins for a few hours, or at worst a few days but, as soon as I come out of the negative emotional state, the goblins lose their internal motor and subside quietly.

It's easy to track the goblins' demise through psychotic episodes. These were goblin driven until 2014 which, instead, was the year of goblins plus black beetles - a new arrival. The black beetles, as I remember, were chiefly a problem at work although the relapse itself was the result of a stressful period at home. The hospital where I worked had, I believed, been invaded by large flying black beetles, which to my puzzlement and distress were being manufactured behind cupboard doors. I knew this was happening because I could hear their wing cases rubbing against their carapaces. There was no obvious logic to this, although unwelcome tiny, black flies intermittently appeared in the office, so perhaps they were the trigger. More problematically from my point of view, these black beetles had also been 'sent' by management to infest my computer. How was I expected to work under this duress and with such compromised equipment? Prudently, unlike during the early days of the goblins, I decided not to ask management this interesting question, and took sick leave until I had a more conventional grasp of reality.

Getting back to work, after this particular episode, was a huge challenge. Occupational health, unsurprisingly, was very cautious and somewhat suspicious of me. Yes, I had the support and input of mental health services but it was my work team leader, L, who made my return possible. She took me out dog walking and asked time and time again why I couldn't go back to work, until I explained to her the black beetle problem which she accepted in a somewhat non-committal way. Then L addressed the issue practically. On several evenings she met me in the hospital's entrance hall - not yet in the general office

- so we could undermine my fears. This was especially kind and thoughtful as she was usually based at another site. I was able to gently reacclimatise myself and, with the help of more medication, accept that the black beetles might be rather less real than I feared.

As a result of this much appreciated and sensible support, I was able to reclaim my now beetle-free computer and continue on at work, in relative tranquillity, until 2020. Dog walking has continued since 2014, and it has, over the years, given me the chance to talk through work anxieties openly in a non-judgemental environment. If things went really wrong I knew the problem would be addressed at work. Like many of my, now ex-colleagues, who have also benefited from her proactive management, I can't thank L enough.

In 2016, I was discharged from mental health services again optimistically believing that everything was now manageable, and I would never need to be referred back. My father was living next door, having moved back from the seaside after the death of my mother, and I had regular support from L. What could possibly go wrong?

2020. The beginning of the coronavirus lockdowns. I didn't consider myself vulnerable, physically or mentally, to the coronavirus germ or the impact of lockdown. My home life was more restricted than usual but not unpleasantly so. I had the company of my father, a garden to look after, my own house and domestic hobbies to enjoy. I continued going to work for the NHS, as usual, and there was no question of me losing my job at any point, although my workload changed as routine operations and procedures were massively curtailed.

My medical records job now required slightly different skills. Previously, I could get away with short bursts of focussed concentration and then a degree of relative mental disengagement. Suddenly, I was being asked to concentrate all day, mostly at a fairly low level but without the recuperative turning off. It quickly mentally exhausted me, particularly as I had to keep the concentration going while listening to a local radio station, with its endless advertisements for skip hire. I really had no need of a skip from twenty miles up the road and would have been happier in a quieter environment. However, my colleagues all preferred working with the radio on. So, I couldn't justifiably complain. 'Anyway, is it such a big deal?' I sensibly asked myself. I'd assimilated changes at work before, as the job had evolved over many years, even though I'd sometimes found them difficult. Work had always been stressful at the best of times, largely because I loathed being constantly assessed and judged.

Even taking these changes into account, why was I so uneasy? There wasn't anything in my work or home life that really matched my rapidly escalating anxiety levels, so I was ashamed of these feelings and wanted to keep them under control. My current life really was better than many. It was a futile ambition as, at some point, although I can't remember the exact moment, my qualitatively normal anxieties tipped from rational to irrational, and trees (of all things) took on a whole new sinister existence.

I didn't have, as far as I remember, a building sense of anxiety about trees themselves; it was more that I experienced a sudden, blinding revelation, a crystal clear new understanding. It was now unequivocally obvious that, of course, I wasn't particularly anxious at all about my current life, so I needn't feel guilty about failing to manage my emotions. No, my unwanted anxieties were all down to trees, my new, previously unsuspected, villainous enemies. In this novel, hastily-constructed world view, trees formed large, powerful networks, with which they ran absolutely everything. My new dictators were also extremely hostile to humans, so very alarming indeed. In a few seconds, I had totally jettisoned a lifetime of belief and experience that trees were just, well, trees. Prior to summer 2020 trees had been entirely neutral. In fact, I liked them; they were a home to birds and other wildlife and generally cheered up, and beautified, the local urban landscape.

I was aware that this tree fear probably didn't happen to everyone but I knew why it had happened to me. During lockdown lunch breaks at work, I sometimes visited a small patch of woodland. This was always a pleasant, calming experience, a place of interlocking flickering patterns of light, birdsong, and the joyful regrowth of late spring and then early summer.

This elysian little patch wasn't much visited by other people and I never felt threatened or anxious there. The only person I really remember was a gentle young man, who'd caught a large rat in a plastic carrying cage (he wasn't sure what it was, but it was definitely a rat) and was releasing it well away from home.

These woodland visits were a new habit, as before lockdown I'd generally walk into the town at lunchtime. Now, I usually rambled about and on sunny days I would briefly sit upon a particular fallen tree. It was this unknowingly dangerous act that had given the trees the opportunity to snare me. Perhaps it was my casual lack of respect, treating the tree as no more than a convenient seat, that had incited this arboreal anger, although I had been totally unaware of any problems at the time.

Scientifically and culturally speaking, I was definitely on sounder ground with trees than I'd been with goblins. Like goblins, trees are part of the natural world. However, unlike goblins, nobody disputes the existence of trees. When trees, out of nowhere, became a problem, it added a new, unfortunate dimension to the situation. Trees must be doing what they're doing because they're real, aren't they? Unlike goblins which are ninety nine percent not real. Self-evident really.

Hence, my new and bizarre tree fantasy had an essentially stable base. I was, also, vaguely aware of recent scientific discoveries. These suggest that trees are essentially social beings, at least with other trees. Quite how aware they are is a subject of ecological discussion. Do trees have an overarching form of consciousness, or are we guilty of anthropomorphism?

They might communicate through fungal networks but it's open to discussion the extent to which such connections are purposeful. That's not for me to determine, but I was vaguely aware of these debates and that, presumably, fuelled my obsession with trees communicating with each other and, to a limited extent, me.

Then there are the symbolic, religious and cultural aspects of trees, going back thousands of years and across the world. I was hardly the first person to recognise the spiritual qualities of trees. Animism is found in many societies and is presumably built into the human psyche. Traditionally, the spirits that inhabit the living world can be malevolent and they may 'need' to be placated. However, recent books, at least in Britain, more often celebrate the miraculous, healing, mindful tree ... definitely not the evil tree. Yet again, when it came to timing, I couldn't be more out of step if I'd tried, with my sudden, pathological obsession; a question of context and degree which was definitely beyond the bounds of my own culturally-accepted normality.

This was problematic, because these new beliefs inspired my leap from, 'I'm very anxious but I shouldn't be,' to, 'those trees are watching me.' But the exact mechanism was, as usual for me, unhappily obscure. I really, really, wish that it wasn't. Yes, I understand that I wriggled out of my uncomfortable emotions by blaming something else, but why did I choose trees and not something more commonly - and currently - seen as threatening, such as 5G radio masts? As I'm not an expert in the workings of the brain, I can work out underlying personal 'whys' for how I might feel or think in a particular way, but I'm not so good at the physical explanation of 'how' it really happens. I could generalise but, as the entire picture is nuanced and not yet fully understood, I won't. Emotionally, I'm guessing that the rising tension and anxiety I experienced at work, a tension and anxiety driven by Covid which affected every part of the NHS, became accidentally associated in my brain with the new experience of visiting woodland at lunchtime.

By the time of the tree episode, I'd had a number of other psychotic episodes so it is easier for me to try and trace the mechanics of this one. Like goblins, there was no obvious reason for trees to be so terrifying. Goblins aren't usually terrifying for people because, although they are famously unpleasant in mythology, grown-ups can generally discount them. Trees, I suppose, could inspire deep anxiety and even fear when their roots undermine the foundations of one's home but, thankfully, that isn't a problem when it comes to my house.

Poor trees are more likely to be accidentally terrifying; it's basically only likely when they themselves come to grief: when they're blown over, or when they lose their branches. I worried about this a lot. Could trees choose to drop limbs on people who'd transgressed? However a tree defines 'transgressed.' When a psychiatrist asked me, 'Why would trees be hostile to humans?' I could only come up with the suggestion that we humans didn't treat trees well; if you're going to imagine a tree as a sentient being, that is a possibility. Therefore, logically speaking, the wooden furnishings at home should have been threatening and I did give some consideration to this point, before concluding they were constructed of dead wood and therefore inert. This was suspiciously handy for me, as I'm not keen on MDF and my furniture is very traditionally wooden. Happily, there was no need to spend hours creating expensive firewood.

There were some obvious similarities with the goblin mythology and, certainly, the trees 'behaved' in a manner that would be familiar to the goblins, even though the details were different. Neither are known for forming evil empires; I was the one who endowed them with this unwarranted capacity. Both were authoritarian, although goblins were more directly controlling of me, reflecting my desperate desire to control and master my life at the time they first appeared. The troublesome trees also emerged at a time of ongoing anxiety and change, but although they did issue commands, these were relatively infrequent, less diverse and less emotionally charged.

Tree commands were largely to do with hanging people, unspecified, from their branches, so the trees had easy access to human life force, or hanging myself from their branches for the same reason. Fortunately, babies were of no interest to the trees at all, perhaps because a baby's potential life force is limited by its size. Although, practically speaking, it would be much easier to hang a small, unresisting body from a tree than an actively dissenting adult.

Thankfully, (especially for those around me), trees could also access human energy without violent input from me. Therefore being too close to trees was highly dangerous, a perpetual risk, as the trees would move millimetres at a time, encroaching on paths when I wasn't looking, and sucking me (and others) spiritually dry. This stolen human energy could replenish itself but, rather like a rechargeable battery, that replenishment was weaker every time, and would then be taken again by a tree or trees. Curiously, I could disrupt this hostile mechanism by standing barefoot next to a spring in a small local stream. Perhaps the spring's inoffensive energy offered an alternative, more friendly version of life. Or maybe I was subconsciously recalling the folklore of healing wells and holy water. As it was summer, my feet didn't get too cold.

I was hyper-conscious of every single tree in the vicinity, even ones which were no more visible than a few twigs on the horizon. My outside universe diminished to 'tree' (vitally important) and 'not tree' (mostly irrelevant). Walks became little more than nervous route marches, accompanied by a dreary, repetitive chant: 'They've moved, yes, they've definitely moved, look away quickly and check again ... They've moved, yes, look away quickly and check again ...' And again. And again. It all seemed very logical. Fruit trees were exempt, as they were busy making fruit, so fortunately eating fruit was permitted which was paradoxical as fruit is, figuratively speaking, stolen from trees. But there again, tree fruit is made to be eaten by predators, whether animal or human, so the tree can proliferate. Not that the trees had me nurturing plum stones, for example, to increase their world domination. On the whole, my trees were more scary than demanding.

There is usually an underlying consistency to a delusional structure. So ... how did this one build? Trees are the largest living thing there is, and size was definitely an issue; broadly speaking the larger the tree, the greater the evil. In a military sense, trees stand about like sentries and the tallest ones could be seen as watchtowers. If such trees were watching me, they were obviously capable of other 'human' characteristics. As I felt generally uneasy, it must be because these humanoid trees, that I was newly aware of, had hostile intent. As trees can communicate with each other (see the science) and they are often found in groupings, from clumps to forests, this hostility could then be multiplied exponentially. Hostility isn't an empty emotion, so the trees must be expressing this malice in some form, the exact extent and methodology of which is unspecified and therefore alarming; by which I mean difficult to categorise and contain, and difficult to submit to reason. If there are millions of trees, which was something I was aware of but hadn't noticed until now, all of which are hostile (or even more emotively evil) and in communication with each other as well, they must be extraordinarily powerful. How could they fuel this powerful network? By taking their energy from humans; that was why I was tired and stressed. Why do trees need all this energy? Because they're secretly running the world. Why is all this extraordinarily dangerous? Because nobody's realised this; they think trees are just trees.

It was my usual egocentric worldview. That's how I got from, 'I'm upset and anxious at work,' (fair enough) via, 'trees are watching me,' (debatable), to, 'evil trees rule the world!' (Totally nuts, but it has just occurred while writing this, that nuts are literally produced by trees, aren't they? I'd better abandon this line of enquiry now.) It's a fairly standard thought process of the paranoid - combining catastrophization with a totally left field point of view.

It made sense - looking at my currently stable home life - that another vortex of anxiety was at work. Initially, inside the hospital was tree free, much as any of us would expect, but as my general anxieties increased, the hospital was invaded and my work computer was, yet again, infected. This was clearly indicated by the usual, and previously innocuous, introduction screen showing a dove with an olive branch. Well, the dove was no problem but that twig it had in its mouth was clearly indicating a tree infestation. I also anxiously watched the cracks in the concrete walls and floors of the hospital, particularly in the basement. This damage was obviously caused by active tree roots: widening, spreading, cracking, crumbling and destroying. The structural instability of the whole building was alarming.

At this point I should add that, whatever I believed at the time, the local hospital is not about to collapse, although I have, over the years, heard rumours that it might be vulnerable to concrete fatigue. There is, however, a metaphor here; as I felt increasingly mentally friable, the physical structure around me was being undermined. Once I took sick leave, the trees at work proliferated, to the extent I couldn't go back to work because I would be suffocated by a room full of mobile, sinister, dead leaves.

Even in the relative safety of home, I couldn't concentrate because my head was full of rustling dead leaves and I could feel the tree roots and filaments sprouting and spreading throughout my body. My sleep was poor (in spite of all the antipsychotic medication), which left me feeling physically unwell. There are quite a number of trees in the local environment and I surreptitiously monitored them through the window, as though I might catch them in some kind of confirmatory evil act when they thought I wasn't really watching.

Oh great.

Going into an episode is terrifying, far more so than in the early days, as I'm now so well aware of what's happening and that awareness is in itself frightening and distressing - quite apart from whichever irrational belief is taking over my life. It's terrifying, as once it gets beyond a certain point (exact moment unspecified, but best described as the moments of revelation), I know I'll uncritically accept all sorts of strange beliefs. Once I've accepted, or created these, it's back down the rabbit hole.

I'll know this really shouldn't be happening, so I'll look for medical help. Other than that anyone who is unfortunate enough to find out what I believe is really going on ('really' being the operative word here, it's 'really' in my world) will have to listen to it anxiously, obsessively and lengthily explained (how to derail my unfortunate GP's evening surgery).

But how ill, or not, did I think I was? Although I sought help, my insight into the situation was definitely compromised. When I spoke to my GP, I begged her not to re-refer me to mental health services. 'Can't you just ask them for advice?' I asked hopefully, totally ignoring government guidelines, which are unequivocal about re-referral to mental health services when there is an inadequate response to medication. How on earth did I think it was realistic to expect a responsible GP to deal with a new psychotic episode on her own?

My GP got round this one by lying gamely, 'They won't say you're ill,' she assured me, clearly having decided thirty seconds into the conversation that the normal rules of engagement didn't apply. So, it was back to childhood again even though it was, admittedly, a therapeutic necessity. Mental health services were in agreement with my GP, describing me in a clinic letter as 'floridly psychotic', the use of the word 'florid' somewhat apposite considering my tree obsession. I bet the psychiatrist enjoyed writing it.

Being at home and unwell wasn't pleasant. I was guilty about not being at work, felt distressed, harassed and frightened, and had the concentration span of a gnat, but was I truly ill? With acres of time on my hands, exacerbated by the practical realities of the coronavirus pandemic, I obsessively researched factitious psychotic disorders, hoping I could properly re-diagnose myself as not psychotic in the least and therefore take control of my life without recourse to the usual antipsychotic medication. I was stalking sanity across the web. It was back to the old optimistic, or perhaps defensive, 'I'm not ill,' although with a great deal less conviction than the early days of my illness. In addition, if I could prove myself not ill, then this would validate the evil tree theory. But did I really want this proven? Yes, it would be reassuring to be right, but then where did it leave me? Surely, it was better to be told I was ill than to face up to the new realities of the evil tree world. As ever, nothing was straightforward.

It was a pointless activity anyway, as everything I read reinforced my unwanted diagnosis, so I continued with antipsychotics as prescribed, augmented by an antidepressant. The only way I could make myself feel better was by wasting hours reading accounts of disasters online, as a sort of grisly reality check. However bad I felt, at least I wasn't being washed away in a tsunami or stranded on Mount Everest. The list goes on. Humanity in general is fragile, not just me.

I was absolutely furious with myself about the tree trouble. Stupid, stupid, stupid. How could I have let this happen? Being ill again was not in my script. That was the past, done, dusted, sorted. It was a double blow; not only had I let myself get ill, but I also looked like a total idiot, yet again. Nobody, when I've enlightened them about any of my delusional constructions, has ever said, 'Yes, that's a really good idea, thank you for bringing it to my attention.' They're usually concerned or amused, or a mixture of the two, and I'm left thinking in the aftermath, 'What just happened? How on earth did I get here?'

After all, I'd been taking 600mg of quetiapine, the antipsychotic, for years and this isn't a low dose. All these years people had been telling me not to mess about with the antipsychotic and this time I genuinely wasn't. I felt cheated. I had also tried to remember and implement all the helpful information and tips I'd received over the last twenty years. However, I had been off antidepressants for a while - my GP was aware and had supported me to try without them - for the record, this was my bright idea, not hers.

Yes, yet again, I'd been misled by stories in the press, this time about the scandal of people taking low doses of antidepressants forever. Do I ever learn? I've never fallen for an online, telephone or general investment scam, but as soon as it comes to mental health I might as well have 'Sucker' stamped on my forehead in fluorescent green. When it came to antidepressants, I was clearly a weak failure unable or unwilling to pull myself together and get on with life. I wilfully over rode the warning bells at the back of my mind: tellingly, these happy, fulfilled antidepressant-free individuals I was reading about didn't seem to have a background of psychosis as well, not at all ... and a psychosis which was, at least partly, driven by the kind of negative emotions that antidepressants help dispel. Maybe my antidepressant experiment would have worked out, as like everyone else, nobody knew that 2020 - and onwards - was going to be so challenging. The one positive of 2020 for me is that neither goblins, trees or anything else have held me responsible for the coronavirus epidemic.

Inevitably, I have, eventually, learnt quite a lot from previous acute episodes, which is useful. So, while this new tree-driven episode was frightening, it was far easier to get over. I've had so much help from professionals, family and friends over the years and I try to keep all of their excellent advice in mind - well, the bits I approve of. I'm not that amenable. I don't argue about medication; I listen to what outsiders tell me; and I remember and try to practise insight. Working on insight, i.e. the whys and wherefores, is hugely important and it's something I can do for myself. I also stick to routines, and that's both physical and mental; get out and about; try to distract myself; and try to maintain a healthy lifestyle. It's all very dull and predictable stuff and it certainly lacks the enticing shiny glamour of the delusional world - but that's only a meretricious, surface glamour, it's quite different actually living there. In addition, I no longer felt compelled to obsessively explore the extent of the tree issue, in a misguided and pointless attempt to take responsibility for it. Instead, I tried to keep in mind the simple question: 'Whatever trees may, or may not, get up to, is it really my problem?'

Then finally, vitally, I also know, which I didn't the first time round, that there is hope and that I will recover, whatever my negative, internal narrative is telling me. I genuinely do want to recover. I'm not interested in being ill; it's frightening, exhausting, bewildering, annoying, humiliating, and ultimately, very, very boring as well. Psychosis is like a self-consuming fire in the brain; it takes everything it can get to feed the flames.

Now I've recovered from the tree episode, I'm careful it doesn't flare up again and at the slightest sign of slippage I warn myself: 'No, whatever you do, just ... don't ... go there.' While writing this, one wet Saturday morning, I bought a clearance copy of a book that usefully summarises various cultural aspects of trees. The information I was reading was hardly groundbreaking and I was already aware of most of it; my background in art history means I have a reasonable grasp of cultural history, especially through visual sources.

As usual, however, it was time for a bit of magical thinking even though I was officially over the tree problem. What was no more than coincidental, I suddenly saw as 'meant'. So, this book, all about trees, was clearly placed at the shop by the trees (precisely how, was not a consideration) as a timely reminder of their power. A sort of sinister 'lest you forget'. Trees would naturally communicate through a book made of that exploited tree product, otherwise known as paper. I needed to know that I was foolishly and wilfully closing my eyes to trees ... and all the rest ... I stamped on this line of enquiry rapidly, but it still left a powerful sense of unease.

My NHS employer's occupational health department had, by this time, been outsourced. When I first called in sick, I was phoned by a pleasant nurse.

'Have you got a diagnosis?' she asked.

'Yes, schizoaffective disorder.' Silence.

'I don't think I know that one,' she said, eventually. 'Do you take any medication for it?'

I named the antidepressant, fine, but she hadn't heard of the antipsychotic quetiapine, even though it's widely prescribed. I'd heard that holding down a normal job with my diagnosis and medication was unusual. Suddenly, I had confirmation.

There was one more occupational health nurse telephone call during the months I was off sick. We went back over the same puzzling ground. (Don't they write it down? Or are they monitoring for inconsistencies in the patient's account?) This time, I was also asked:

'And what would you say was the main reason for you not being able to go to work?'

It was my turn for a long silence. Even though I'd entirely forgotten the interview with the occupational health doctor, back when I was a museum curator - the one recorded in my hospital notes where I'd mentioned the need to monitor goblins in the Art Store - I knew better than to mention my workplace tree infestation. Telling the truth, however, was an ordeal and my chest was tight with anxiety. It meant denying the reality of the evil trees, which felt irresponsible and dangerous. Eventually, I took a deep breath and said, uncertainly,

'Psychosis, I guess.'

This was, for me, a huge admission as I was no longer taking refuge in the delusionally unanswerable. It had been a long journey.

'Oh, bless,' said the nurse kindly, and from that point her team showed no further desire to talk to me at all, not that I asked. If you want to get occupational health off your back, psychosis is a good ailment to choose. You don't need to bother with the details.

This time, I know I recovered more quickly from the tree episode because I chose to leave my NHS job. Leaving work was my decision. I wasn't pressured to do so by my manager, in fact I was asked to reconsider my decision. Reconsider? I can't convey what a huge boost to my confidence this was. I was quite touched. I thought they'd be glad to see the back of me but they obviously thought I was a reasonable member of the team. My father commented that perhaps because of my 'condition' (his choice of word), I might sometimes think that my colleagues were more hostile to me than they actually were ... I know I could have gone back to work, but it would have been a huge effort, and I'd got to the stage where I could just about fund myself, without claiming benefits, so my self-respect remained intact.

I don't miss working at all, particularly the effort it took to keep my mind on the job, and also the stress of being answerable to other people. I know this is bizarre; I have a history of authoritarian delusions of control, carefully constructed to bully me and boss me about, and I really don't like being told what to do.

Admittedly, leaving work was key to my discharge from mental health services. If I'd tried to get back to work I would have needed more support. I was discharged in spring 2021, after about eight months. It was a perfectly amicable split as I'd made it clear, right from my re-referral, that I wanted to get back to GP care as soon as possible. I'd actually been offered more support from mental health services than I wanted; I suspect my enthusiasm for discharge was, at least at the beginning, seen as a lack of insight. They were probably right. The web is full of people complaining about being discharged from mental health services when they're still ill (or even worse, struggling to get help at all). The reverse problem is much rarer.

Crucially important, also, was my more grown-up response to my illness. Once I'd finally (mostly) shed trees, it was clear to me that after the first few unhinged months, with help, I could get on top of things and move on with my life. It was something that I would never have imagined in the darkest, goblin days. 'Evil' trees, thanks to their relatively brief spell in the ascendancy, have left far less troublesome traces in my brain.

My story is full of reasons to be grateful … There are so many. I started enumerating them, and more importantly believing them, the day I first stood in Coventry Cathedral; one of Britain's favourite modernist buildings. When was it? 2006? Perhaps. Sunlight shone through the immense, stained glass windows and coloured the paving and me. It was quiet, and I was able to stand alone, and let the light flow over me. Colours pulsed in my fingers, my heart and my brain, coursing joyfully throughout my whole body. If I were religious I would have called it the light of heaven, but as I'm not, I'll describe the windows as a sublime moment of human creation. The effect was the same. I felt for the first time for years that perhaps life could get better. There was still beauty in life, in all its forms, provided I was prepared to look for it and, most of all, acknowledge it.

I feel privileged that my life was given back to me. I've been invariably supported by my family and friends, and by many, many people in the NHS. It could have been so much worse. I know I'll never get myself back fully but it's a recovery that allows me to have a reasonable quality of life. Mine is not a story of triumph (I wish …) more a story of building resilience, and coming to terms with my illness.

But I have to be honest. I've watched with envy as my friends have settled down, had children, got on with their careers and all the rest. What have I achieved? If I look dispassionately at my life, I've achieved nothing much since the age of thirty. After that, it's been one long regression, both personally and professionally.

Having a brain you can't trust isn't an easy thing to live with. Will it happen again? When will the normal stresses and strains of life send me off into a weird world? I hope it won't happen again but I feel physically sick at the thought. What will it be next time? Partridges, unicorns, daisies? Who's to say? I like Surrealist art, but I don't want to live in it. Yes I know, whatever happens, I will get better, but psychosis fundamentally undermines my concept of who I really am. When that goes, who are you really?

Acknowledgements

First of all I'd like to thank my family and friends, who are a faithful lot, all things considered, and cheerfully put up with my peculiarities. Without their continuing love and support, this book would never have been written. I won't name you here, but you know who you are.

From a book perspective, special thanks to:

Dr Karen Wright, Professor of Nursing at the University of Central Lancashire, who initially encouraged me to share my experiences as other people might find them useful, and also generously read and commented on this text during the writing process. She is a great educator and encourager of many, not just me.
Hilary Machell, old friend and freelance cultural fundraiser, marketer and writer, FRSA member (see Hilary Machell on twitter) who not only read and warmly commented on this book, but also proofread it and corrected my grammar. As I made some alterations to the text after proofing, I take full responsibility for any remaining textual errors.
Alex Walker and Liz Mitchell, old friends who generously read this book not long before completion, and offered their memories and encouragement.
'Sean' who I had brief contact with through social media while writing this book, and, kindly read chapter 1 before giving me the go ahead.

Jane Chisholm, former NHS psychiatric nurse. I have had no contact with her after she retired from local mental health services. Although she appears very briefly in this book, she worked with me on and off over ten years, and gave me far more than I can convey.
Lisa Williams, whose long term workplace (and personal support) helped me retain my NHS job for many years. Without Jane and Lisa's long term input, I might never have been confident and insightful enough to write this book.

Printed in Great Britain
by Amazon

81922908R00130